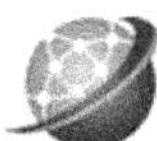

Dedicated to All Safety, Health and Environmental Professionals

Striving to Protect

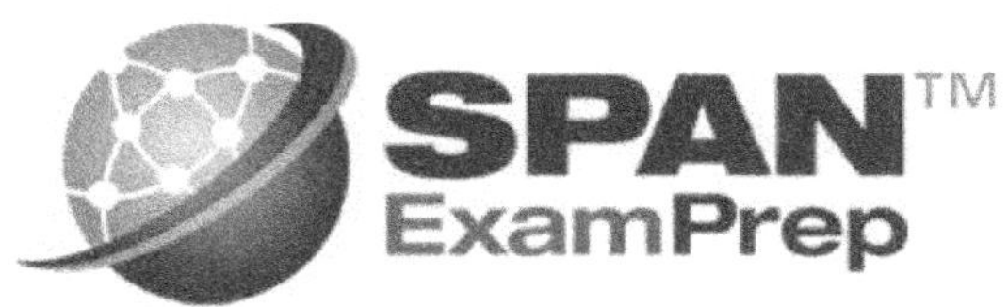

This publication is not intended to guarantee that the user will pass an exam, become certified or in general may not cover every aspect of the certification process.

The information contained in this study workbook is intended to be used in preparation for the Associate Safety Professional examination and should not be used as an authority in the professional practice of safety, health, or environmental compliance.

The Safety Management Specialist® (SMS®) Certification is a registered trademark of the Board of Certified Safety Professionals (BCSP).
The opinions expressed are those of the authors and no guarantee, warranty, or other representation is made as to the absolute correctness or sufficiency of any information contained in this study workbook.

Daniel J. Snyder, Ed.D, CSP, SMS

402 W. Mt Vernon St #111
Nixa, Missouri 65714
www.spansafety.com

ISBN 978-1-886786-36-3 **(set)**
ISBN 978-1-886786-34-9 **(v.1)**
ISBN 978-1-886786-35-6 **(v.2)**

Table of Contents

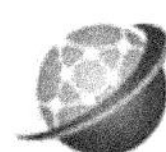

Introduction

There are two major objectives of this study materials:

1) Provide candidates the knowledge and skills to successfully attain Safety Management Specialist® (SMS) certification.
2) Enhance skills, knowledge and abilities as a safety professional.

This workbook is designed to be used as a resource for self-directed study in preparation for the SMS exam. In the fast track three-day workshop conducted by SPAN™ Safety Workshops, participants are provided expert guidance and use the same content presented in these workbooks. This curriculum is also used in the SPAN™ CertBok® Exam Prep Online Learning Management System (LMS).

Workshops are conducted periodically throughout the year so that professionals can take the examination as soon as they are prepared. Visit the SPAN™ website for workshop dates and locations. www.spansafety.com

The exam is designed for candidates with ten years of professional safety experience. Generally, it takes the average safety and health practitioner about 40-60 hours of dedicated self-study, in addition to a workshop, to adequately prepare for the examination. The self-study can generally be accomplished in about 4 to 12 weeks.

The workbook is divided into two volumes designed for self-study and facilitated professional development workshops. After each section of the workbook there are fully developed explanations for the answer selected for each question. In many cases information about all selections offered as possible answers will be included to assist in developing a better understanding of the subject. These sessions are designed to allow the safety professional to measure progress during the extended program of self-study that is normally required to pass the certification exams.

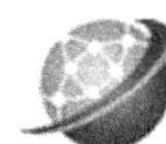

Considerable effort has been made to fully develop and explain the concepts and techniques discussed. However, given the differences in the background and experience of the safety practitioners sitting for the SMS examination, it is impossible to explain all concepts to all candidates. The materials are based on the exam blueprint and subject matter expertise.

Browse through the rest of the first volume, stopping and reading whenever a subject or question is of interest. Study explanations to all questions as these represent much of the exam philosophy and may add significant value to candidates' test preparation. These are only suggestions.

After reviewing the workbook, establish a study plan. There are voluminous resources available for each domain of the exam blueprint. Simply stated, chance favors the prepared mind and candidates should have a study plan. Budget adequate time to master the material.

This workbook is designed to optimize study time. There is no extraneous or "nice to know" information in this workbook. All the information is important. Concentrating on the areas emphasized in the text should reduce research and study time considerably.

The BCSP exams have changed very dramatically in the past few years and SPAN™ conducts ongoing research and development to ensure accuracy and quality of curriculum based on the actual exam blueprint. ***This workbook does not contain actual SMS test questions*** and uses a question and answer format with detailed explanations. Difficult concepts or theories may have material presented in a table, diagram, illustration, or a paraphrased format. This method is used to allow broad coverage of the material and optimize study efforts.

The beginning sections of the workbook are devoted to enhancing knowledge and skills in:

- The exam process
- Study and testing techniques

Content may serve as preliminary exercises to engage the analytical portions of the brain and help prepare candidates for the mathematical components of the exam. The problems are representative of the exam based on the blueprint.

From the introductory sections, the workbook progresses to individual areas on each of the nine SMS exam blueprint domains. These nine blueprint domains utilize the question and answer format designed to mimic the type of questions offered on the exam. Explanations are offered to reduce research time considering the examination covers a tremendous amount of subject matter.

The questions presented are representative of the questions found on the actual examination(s). For this reason, candidates must understand the area (areas) to which the question is pertaining. Many times, this will require additional study. However, do not stray too far from the subject or direction and focus will be lost. Follow what the workbook attempts to provide.

An estimated 65% of the scored questions must be answered correctly to pass the SMS examination. Mastery of the concepts contained herein. Become familiar with the subject areas contained in the workbooks through repetition will help to identify areas of strength and weakness unique to every individual

The assumption is made that only fully qualified safety practitioners will attempt to sit for the SMS examination, which means everyone using this workbook has a solid foundation in the Safety and Health field. Given this assumption, no attempt has been made to provide a basic safety text. Rather, the problems presented in this book are representative of questions that may be expected to appear on the SMS examination and based on the exam blueprint. The workbook is designed as a guide and depending upon an individual's knowledge baseline, additional research may be required.

The challenge of achieving certification is a difficult task. Embrace the journey of professional development in preparation for the exam. The modern safety professional must be an adaptive leader and lifelong learner.

This curriculum has been carefully checked for accuracy, but errors may exist. Should and an error be discovered, contact the author via info@spansafetyworkshops.com

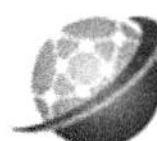

Safety Management Specialist (SMS) Workshop Lesson Plan

Course Description:

The primary purpose of the SPAN™ three-day SMS exam prep workshop is to assist safety professionals to successfully pass the Board of Certified Safety Professional's (BCSP) SMS exam. This is a fast pace agenda, and most will require additional study to be successful on the SMS exam. The SMS workshop is scheduled from 8am until 4:00pm daily with breaks and lunch on your own. The facilitator is an experienced practitioner and subject matter expert on the exam blueprint domains. Learning strategies include lecture, guided discussion, case studies, self-directed learning, and learner discovery methods.

Orientation/Rules:

- Emergency Exits
- Restrooms
- Breaks
- Silence phones, lap-tops, anything that makes a sound
- We are all adult learners and professionals
- No pictures, audio or video recording
- Ask Questions
- Participate in discussions

Course Objectives:

At the completion of this workshop participants will be able to:

- Describe SMS exam requirements.
- Determine the level of difficulty for the "SMS" exam.
- Review problems aligned with competencies outlined in the exam blueprint
- Analyze your knowledge gaps
- Locate reference materials to enhance knowledge
- Establish a study plan

SMS Workshop Schedule

Day 1	Time
Introduction (Purpose & Objectives)	0800
Personnel Introductions	
The SMS Examination Blueprint	
Study planning, testing strategies, exam philosophy	
Break	0930-0945
Domain 1: Management Systems	
Lunch on your own	1130-1230
Domain 1: Management Systems	
Break	1400
Domain 1: Management Systems	
Adjourn	1600
Day 2	**Time**
Domain 2: Risk Management	0800
Break	0930-0945
Domain 2: Risk Management	
Lunch on your own	1130-1230
Domain 3: Safety Health & Environmental Concepts	
Break	1400-1415
Domain 3: Safety Health & Environmental Concepts	
Adjourn	1600
Day 3	**Time**
Domain 4: Incident Investigation and Emergency Preparedness	0800
Break	0930-0945
Domain 4: Incident Investigation and Emergency Preparedness	
Lunch on your own	1130-1230
Domain 5: Business Case of Safety	
Break	1400-1415
Domain 5: Business Case of Safety	
Closing discussion	1500
Adjourn	1600

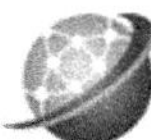

BCSP Certification Matrix

	CSP	ASP	GSP	SMS	OHST	CHST	STS/ STSC	CET
Minimum Education	Bachelor's degree[1] or Associate's degree[2]	Bachelor's degree or Associate degree	Bachelor's or Master's degree [3]	High School Diploma or GED	High School Diploma or GED	High School Diploma or GED	**N/A**	High School Diploma or GED
Minimum Training	**N/A**[4]	**N/A**	**N/A**	**N/A**	**N/A**	**N/A**	30 hours of SH&E[5] training	Delivery of 135 hours of training[6]
Minimum Work Experience	4 years of experience[7] **And** Hold an authorized credential[8]	1 year of experience[9]	No experience required[10]	10 years of safety management related experience[11]	3 years of experience[12]	3 years of construction experience[13]	2 years supervisory experience[14] Or 4 years' work experience	Hold an authorized credential.[15]
Application Fees	$160	$160	**N/A**	$160	$140	$140	$120	$140
Examination Fees	$350	$350	**N/A**	$350	$300	$300	$185	$300
Eligibility Extension Fees	$100	$100	**N/A**	$100	$100	$100	$100	$100
Renewal Fees	$150	$140	$140	$140	$120	$120	$60	$120
Passing Scores	100/175 57%	107/175 61%	**N/A**	106/175 60.5%	116/175 66.2%	108/175 61.7%	**STS:** 61/87 70.1% **STSC:** 60/87 68.9%	119/175 68%
Recertification *(5-year cycle)*	25 points	25 points	**N/A**	25 points	20 points	20 points	30 hours of safety and health courses[16]	20 points[17]

[1] In any field
[2] In a safety and health or related field
[3] from an ABETASAC or AABI accredited QAP program
[4] Not Applicable
[5] Safety, Health and Environmental
[6] In safety, health and environmental-related areas
[7] Where safety is at least 50%, preventative, professional level with breadth and depth of safety duties
[8] ASP, CIH, CMIOSH, CRSP, GSP, SISO, NEBOSH National or International Diploma in Occupational Health and Safety, Diploma in Industrial Safety from CLI/RLIs of the Government of India
[9] Where safety is at least 50%, preventative, professional level with breadth and depth of safety duties
[10] Must achieve the CSP within eligibility period once CSP experience requirement is met
[11] A minimum of 35% of the job tasks must be related to management of safety related programs, processes, procedures, personnel, etc.)
[12] At least 35% of primary job duties involve safety and health
[13] At least 35% of primary job duties involve safety and health
[14] Related to the STS industry exam for which candidate is applying (work experience must be a minimum part time [18 hrs./week] to qualify)
[15] ASP, CDGP, CFPS CHMM, CHST, CIH, CMIOSH, CRSP, CSP, OHST, STS, or STSC
[16] Or by retaking the STS/STSC exam or earning the OHST, CHST, ASP or CSP
[17] With 2.8 of these points in attending a training, development or instructional technology class

About the SMS Exam

Shortly after the turn of the century there began appearing in this country, persons practicing the art and science of safety work. These practitioners came from different academic backgrounds and had a multitude of work experience ranging from operations to engineering. They all had one common goal, promoting the safety and health of employees.

One must have 10 years of experience before achieving the Safety Management Specialist® (SMS) designation, which is the Gold Standard in safety certification.

The BSCP was chartered by the American Society of Safety Engineers (ASSE) in 1969, to establish a method of measuring qualifications for the safety profession. The Board established qualification standards and began issuing certification shortly after being founding. Although chartered as an independent, separately-incorporated board, the BCSP has several sponsoring organizations which provide members to the BCSP Board of Directors. These sponsoring organizations are as follows:

- American Society of Safety Engineers (ASSE)
- American Industrial Hygiene Association (AIHA)
- National Safety Council (NSC)
- Institute of Industrial Engineers (IIE)
- Society of Fire Protection Engineers (SFPE)
- International System Safety Society (ISSS)
- National Fire Protection Association (NFPA)
- National Environmental Training Association (NESHTA)

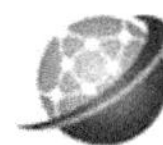

The BCSP's certifications are accredited by independent, third-party organizations that regularly evaluate certification requirements. Accreditation assures:

- Governance
  - Nominations/elections
  - Peer participation
  - Public participation
- Financial disclosure
  - Stability and financial condition
  - Budget details
- Fairness to candidates
- Examinations
  - Validity
  - Reliability
  - Passing scores
- Recertification
- Independence from preparation
- Management systems

International Accreditation is provided by the American National Standards Institute (ANSI 17024/ISO)[18]. National Accreditation is achieved through both the National Commission for Certifying Agencies (NCCA)[19] and the Council of Engineering and Scientific Specialty Boards (CESB)[20].

[18] ASP, CSP
[19] ASP, CSP, OHST, CHST, STS
[20] CET

Accredited Certification vs. Certificate Program

Accredited Certification	Certificate Program
Results from an assessment process	Results from an educational process
Typically requires some amount of professional experience	For novice and experienced professionals
Awarded by a third-party, standard-setting organization	Awarded by training and educational programs or institutions
Indicates master/competency as measured against a defensible set of standards, usually by application or exam	Indicates completion of a course or series of courses with a specific focus; is different than a degree granting program
Standards set through a defensible, industry-wide process (job analysis/role delineation) that results in an outline of required knowledge and skills	Course content set a variety of ways (faculty committee; dean; instructor; occasionally though defensible analysis of topic care)
Typically results in a designation to use after one's name; may result in a document to hang on the wall or keep in a wallet	Usually listed on a resume detailing education; may result in a document to hang on the wall
Has on-going requirements to maintain; individual must demonstrate knowledge of content; holder must demonstrate he/she continues to meet requirements	Is the end result; individual may or may not demonstrate knowledge of course content at the end of a set period in time

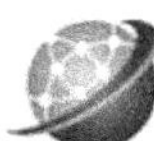

Benefits of Certification

The process of certification commands a considerable amount of effort. Many safety practitioners wonder if the advantages of certification justify all the effort. The primary advantage of certification is that it provides a credential. The SMS indicates that a safety professional has achieved a standard level of qualification as judged by their professional peers. This level of qualification is important in establishing credibility within the ever-growing field of Safety, Health and Environment (SH&E). Employment opportunities are much greater for personnel holding SMS certification, the courts recognize the certification as a step toward authentication as an expert witness, and it is almost always required to do consultant work in the field of safety today. There are several reasons that should cause candidates to think about starting the process of obtaining certification *right now.*

- A growing trend by states to license safety professionals, much like physicians, engineers, architects, and other professionals. Some states have that authority under their duty to "protect the health, safety and welfare of the public."

- Substantial support to modify existing safety and health laws to acknowledge certified "safety specialists". Some projects require a certified professional to be on staff.

- Certified Safety and Health professionals obtain employment earlier and receive greater compensation than non-certified employees.

- As the requirements increase, the examinations may become even more dynamic, complex, difficult to pass and expensive, both in time and financial investments.

These and other recent developments add up to a future environment where a certification is going to be the desired/required credential. Being an SMS will become much more important, more lucrative, and more difficult to obtain. Like the other professional certification/registration examinations, the SMS exam helps to advance your career path.

Overview of the SMS Certification Process

The following information concerning the requirements for certification may have changed after publication. It is strongly suggested candidates contact the BCSP for current information. For exact requirements, go to the BCSP web site at www.bcsp.org and review the SMS complete guide. There are common questions by potential candidates such as "What do I have to do to get the SMS?"

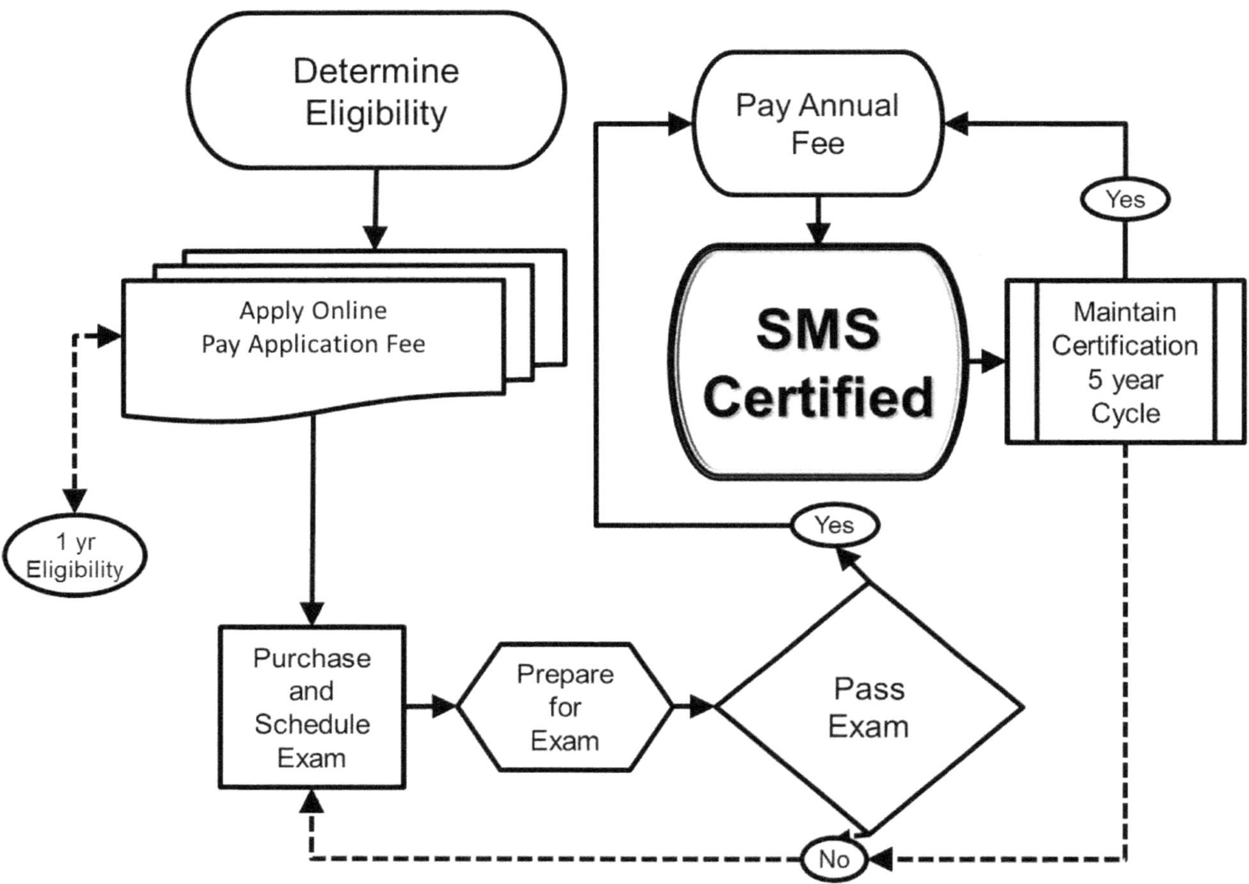

The SMS is a certification awarded by BCSP to individuals who meet all the requirements established by the Board. Along with the education and experience requirements, candidates must successfully complete the examinations.

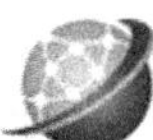

SMS Qualifications

- Qualifying Criteria for Experience
    - Ten years of professional experience
    - Professional safety is primary function ($\geq$ 35% of position)
    - Primary responsibility must be the prevention of harm to people, property, or the environment
    - Must be at professional level (responsible charge)
    - Breadth: Safety Tasks, Hazard Types, etc.
- Pass the SMS examinations leading to the SMS certification
- Recertification Requirements:
    - 25 Points Every 5 Years
    - 10 Point Categories (Some with Point Limitations)
    - Practice
    - Membership
    - Service
    - Publishing, Presenting, Patents
    - Writing Exam Questions
    - Professional Development Conferences
    - Safety-Related Courses, Seminars, Quizzes
    - Continuing Education
    - New Advanced Degree
    - Other Certifications/Re-Examination

A candidate for certification may take the SMS exam after meeting the academic/experience requirements. The SMS is truly a comprehensive practice test. It covers the applied knowledge expected of a safety professional at the practitioner level.

Before taking the SMS Exam, the academic/experience requirements must be met, the candidate must have ten years of acceptable professional safety experience. When a candidate has successfully completed the Safety Management Specialist Examination, they are designated a "Safety Management Specialist®" (SMS).

The entire process of certification generally takes from 3 to 6 months, allowing plenty of time to **PLAN** an individual study program. Costs associated with the certification process are as follows:

SMS Criteria	
Training Prerequisite	N/A
Work Experience	At least 10 years of experience where safety is at least 35%, preventative, professional level with breadth and depth of safety duties
Application Fees	$160
Examination Fees	$350
Eligibility Extension Fees	$100
Renewal Fees	$140
Passing Scores	TBD
Recertification (5-year cycle)	25 points

The above information is accurate as of this printing. For more current information, candidates should contact the Board at:

Board of Certified Safety Professionals
8645 Guion Road
Indianapolis, IN 64268
Phone (317) 593-4800
Fax (317) 593-4400
www.bcsp.org

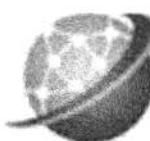

The SMS Examination Blueprint

Effective as of 2017

Domain	Weight
Domain 1: Management Systems	20%
Domain 2: Risk Management	17.1%
Domain 3: Safety, Health and Environmental Concepts	33.1%
Domain 4: Incident Investigation and Emergency Preparedness	11.5%
Domain 5: Business Case of Safety	18.3%

The Safety Management Specialist (SMS) examination is designed to test applied knowledge and the application of experience gained through professional practice. The computerized beta test consists of 200 questions. Candidates are allowed 4.5 consecutive hours to complete all questions. Laminated scratch paper and a marker will be provided by the testing service. After finishing the computerized examination, a pass-fail grade will be given. A detailed score report will be mailed later from the BCSP if a candidate fails the exam. As of this printing, the SMS passing score is yet to be determined.

Domain 1: Management Systems 20%
Knowledge of: 1. Principles and common elements of safety management systems (e.g., continuous improvement, safety processes, controls, measurement, standards, implementation) 2. Principles and techniques for encouraging employee involvement and commitment (e.g., value-based safety) 3. Principles and techniques for encouraging management commitment to safety (e.g., voluntary protection program (VPP), mission statement, management involvement in jobsite assessment) 4. Techniques and principles for goal setting (e.g., SMART) 5. Principles and techniques of internal audits 6. Competency/skills assessment management systems (e.g., new hire orientation, assurance of experience, job skills, on the job training) as it pertains to worker safety 7. General concepts of effective trainings (e.g., learning retention, adult learning principles, training delivery) 8. Recordkeeping related to training and education (e.g., annual, one-time, recertification or retraining) 9. Management of corrective actions (e.g., follow up, follow through, closure of actions, time periods, tracking corrective actions) 10. Unsafe conditions and acts and how they relate to incidents (e.g., Swiss cheese model, bowtie model) 11. Management of change (MOC) procedure and organizational change process 12. Common elements of contractor or multi-employer worksite safety programs (e.g., prequalification, selecting, monitoring, managing risk between contractor and host)
Skill to: 1. Recognize leading and lagging indicators 2. Set and prioritize safety-related goals 3. Assess training needs (regulatory and risk-based)

Domain 2: Risk Management 17.1%

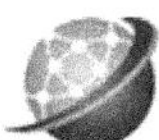

Knowledge of: 1. Resources for hazard prevention and control management (e.g., external resources, internal resources, industry standards, subject matter experts) 2. Work planning and controls (e.g., job safety analysis, preliminary hazard analysis, job/task hazard analysis, safe work permit) 3. Prevention through Design concepts (e.g., managing safety through the lifecycle of the program) 4. Common liability exposures (e.g., tort, joint liability, attractive nuisance) 5. Common types of insurance coverage (e.g., differences between property and liability coverage) 6. Hierarchy of controls (e.g., elimination, engineering, substitutions)
Skill to: 1. Interpret and apply information related to hazard prevention and control management (e.g., internal resources, external resources, industry standards, safety data sheet) 2. Identify safety, health, and environmental risk (e.g., checklists, brainstorming, observation, lessons learned, experience, HAZID, process safety) 3. Analyze safety, health, and environmental risk (e.g., severity and likelihood/frequency matrix, historical information, industry data, "what if" analysis, process safety) 4. Evaluate and prioritize safety, health, and environmental risk (e.g., high/low risk) 5. Review and refine implemented safety, health, environmental controls to ensure they are effective 6. Use a risk matrix 7. Apply the hierarchy of controls to various types of hazards while considering the likelihood and severity

Domain 3: Safety, Health, and Environmental Concepts 33.1%

Knowledge of:

1. Concepts in the Globally Harmonized System of Classification and Labeling of Chemicals (GHS)
2. Common controls for slips, trips, and falls (from all levels)
3. Common controls for working with electricity
4. Common controls for working in confined spaces
5. Common controls for working around machinery and equipment
6. Common controls for bloodborne pathogens
7. Common controls for lead
8. Common controls for asbestos
9. Common controls for radiation (ionizing and non-ionizing)
10. Common controls for temperature extremes (e.g., cold or heat stress, contact with extreme temperatures, thermal stress)
11. Common controls for vibration (e.g., whole body, hand/arm)
12. Common controls for noise
13. Common controls for ergonomic hazards associated with the type of work, body positions, or strain on the body from working conditions (e.g., improperly adjusted workstations/chairs, frequent lifting, awkward movements, poor posture, repetitive movements, use of too much force, compression)
14. Common controls for any form of chemical hazards (e.g., liquids, vapors, fumes, dusts, gases, flammable liquids, and pesticides)
15. Common controls for workplace stressors (e.g., workload demand, fatigue, harassment, lack of schedule flexibility, lack of control)
16. Occupational health programs (e.g., medical surveillance, fit for duty, return to work, substance abuse testing)

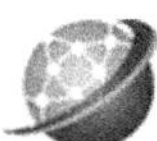

Skill to:

1. Recognize unsafe conditions or acts that can cause slips, trips, and falls (from all levels)
2. Recognize unsafe conditions or acts when working with electricity
3. Recognize unsafe conditions or acts when working in confined spaces
4. Recognize unsafe conditions or acts when working around machinery and equipment (e.g., caught in, struck by, pinch points)
5. Recognize conditions that could lead to unsafe exposures to molds and allergens
6. Recognize unsafe conditions or acts related to potential exposures to bloodborne pathogens
7. Recognize unsafe conditions or acts related to potential exposures lead
8. Recognize unsafe conditions or acts related to potential exposures to asbestos
9. Recognize unsafe conditions or acts related to potential exposures to radiation (ionizing and non-ionizing)
10. Recognize unsafe conditions or acts related to potential exposures to temperature extremes (e.g., cold or heat stress, contact with extreme temperatures, thermal stress)
11. Recognize unsafe conditions or acts related to potential exposures to vibration (e.g., whole body, hand/arm)
12. Recognize unsafe conditions or acts related to potential exposures to noise
13. Recognize unsafe conditions or acts related to ergonomic hazards associated with the type of work, body positions, or strain on the body from working conditions (e.g., improperly adjusted workstations/chairs, frequent lifting, awkward movements, poor posture, repetitive movements, use of too much force, compression)
14. Recognize unsafe conditions or acts related to exposures to any form of chemicals (e.g., liquids, vapors, fumes, dusts, gases, flammable liquids, and pesticides)
15. Recognize unsafe conditions or acts related to workplace stressors (e.g., workload demand, fatigue, harassment, lack of schedule flexibility, lack of control)

Domain 4: Incident Investigation and Emergency Preparedness 11.5%
Knowledge of: 1. Fundamentals of causal analysis (e.g., 5 whys, root cause analysis) 2. Components or elements of an effective incident/accident management program 3. Emergency action requirements/procedures (e.g., response plans, evacuations, preparedness, operation upsets) 4. Components or elements of an emergency response plan (e.g., roles and responsibilities, emergency contact information, stakeholder notification, media response) 5. Incident command structure in emergency response 6. Techniques for identifying gaps in an emergency response plan (e.g., table top drills, lessons learned) 7. Basic elements of workers' compensation and case management programs
Skill to: 1. Calculate incident and injury rates

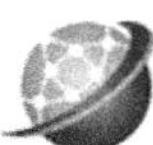

Domain 5: Business Case of Safety 18.3%

Knowledge of:

1. Cost/benefit analysis principles and common techniques (e.g., return on investment [ROI], as low as reasonably practicable [ALARP], as low as reasonably achievable [ALARA])
2. Direct and indirect costs in relation to safety
3. Experience modification rate (EMR), or premium rate, and how it is used
4. Principles of positive safety/organizational culture and common techniques for creating a positive safety culture (e.g., Hearts & Minds, behavioral safety management [BSM], behavior-based safety [BBS], stop work, open communication, culture or perception surveys)
5. Indicators of a positive safety/organizational culture (e.g., leading indicators, management system, management commitment)
6. Techniques and processes for communicating hazards and controls to stakeholders (e.g., management, workforce)
7. Presentation techniques or best practices for communicating technical and other safety information to stakeholders (e.g., management, workforce)
8. Conflict management techniques (e.g., situational leadership, good conflict versus bad conflict, diffusion techniques, relationship management)
9. Common leadership strategies or principles (e.g., setting good example, building trust)
10. BCSP Code of Ethics

Skill to:

1. Interpret cost/benefit analysis
2. Interpret leading and lagging indicators (e.g., training metrics, safety initiatives, incident and injury rates)
3. Develop a safety business case for additional budget, resources, other support, etc. (e.g., use financial tools to make a case for investing in safety program or initiative)
4. Communicate safety on multi-employer/contractor worksites
5. Facilitate or lead safety meetings (e.g., agenda, review safety plans, safety stand-down, shift handover)
6. Communicate (internal) safety activities and performance (e.g., reports, initiatives, lessons learned, requirements) to management and personnel
7. Communicate (external) safety risks and performance information (e.g., reports, presentations, risk/incident plans) to key stakeholders (e.g., public safety organizations, regulatory agencies, community)
8. Write communications that promote safety objectives and activities (e.g., safety proposal development, risk management plans, noncompliance response)

Taking the Computer Based Exam

One major goal of the BCSP is to offer certification examinations with a high degree of validity and reliability to promote a fair assessment of a candidate's competency as a safety and health practitioner.

Testing on computer is done via Pearson VUE (www.pearsonvue.com) Examinations can be taken every business day at many locations throughout the world. Many locations also have evening and Saturday hours.

Candidates must complete an application and return it, supporting information and application fee ($160) to the Board of Certified Safety Professionals (BCSP). Once a candidate has been approved and has paid the examination fee ($350), the Board will mail an examination authorization letter. Once the application is approved, candidates have 1 year to arrange for an actual examination date. Arrangements are made directly with Pearson VUE via on-line or via the national toll-free number **888.269.2219**. Some Pearson VUE Testing Centers are busier than others, so schedule early if possible.

At the Pearson VUE centers, a candidate signs in, presents identifications and is seated at a computer workstation. The center provides laminated graph paper and a marker. There is a short orientation and practice program to acquaint candidates with the examination procedure. During actual testing a small clock in the monitor screen corner keeps track of the remaining time.

ABSOLUTELY NO NOTES OR REFERENCE MATERIALS ARE ALLOWED! Laminated graphing paper and writing utensils will be provided. After finishing the computerized examination, a pass-fail grade will be given. A detailed score report will be mailed later from the BCSP.

For worldwide locations, look at the web site www.pearsonvue.com.

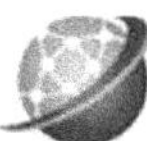

Frequently Asked Questions about the Computer Exam

NOTE: Remember the best and most current source of information on procedures and policies for the computer test is directly from the BCSP at (317) 593-4800 and www.bcsp.org.

Question — How do the questions appear on the computer screen? How do I make answer selections? Can I back up or mark questions so that I can come back to them? Do I need to be a computer whiz to take this test?

Answer — Examination questions appear one at a time and look similar to the questions in the workbook. With a mouse or keys, the candidate selects the preferred answer and moves on to the next question. Questions may be marked for further review or skipped and revisited later. After the last question, a list appears and shows item numbers, answers selected, and questions marked or skipped. Since the computer test is very "friendly" candidates do not have to be computer literate to take this exam.

Question — Can you bring food or drinks into the exam room?

Answer — No. All candidates are given a small locker for personal belongings, including snacks, purses, watches, etc. Access to this locker may or may not be allowed depending upon the testing center.

Question — What can I take into the exam room?

Answer — ID cards are permitted. Everything else must go into personal lockers.

Question — What is furnished in the exam cubicle?

Answer — One laminated sheet of paper, one marker and the computer monitor, keyboard and mouse.

Question What is the workstation/cubicle like?

Answer It is generally very nice, although this may vary with different Pearson VUE Centers. Cubicles are large, with a desktop about 3'x 4', excellent lighting, in a very quiet setting, with comfortable, padded adjustable chairs. The keyboard and mouse take up all space in front of the monitor, so calculations must be done off to the side.

Question Are there any children in the exam room?

Answer No. The room is for adult testing only. All children activities are in separate areas of the Pearson VUE Center.

Question How many other people are in the room?

Answer There are multiple workstations in the exam room. The number of people varies with time and day. The proctor has a view of the entire room via glass window and corner mirrors on the ceiling. Testing is also taped by video and audio monitoring.

Question Can I take breaks?

Answer Yes, as many and as often as necessary. However, the clock keeps running and signing out is required each time, along with a finger print check.

Question Do I need ID's?

Answer One ID with photo and signature is mandatory. Photograph and a finger print are done during sign-in.

Question Do I need my Authorization letter with Candidate ID Number?

Answer This letter is usually not required, but it is advised to take it just in case. The ID number is always needed when scheduling examination appointments.

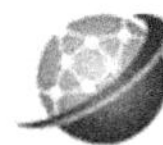

Question Can I schedule the exam any time?

Answer No. Certain times are designated for professional exams. Book testing slot several weeks in advance to secure the desired time and day.

Question Is there enough time to finish the exam?

Answer This is very subjective. Most candidates have found there was plenty of time to finish testing and have adequate review time, but other people did not finish in the allotted time. The time per question (1.5 minutes) is the same as the written exam and the authors found the computer not to be a factor in this area.

Question Are there graphs to interpret? How are clear are the graphics?

Answer Yes, there are a limited number of graphs to read. They are a little harder to read on the screen, but not significantly. Graphics are quite acceptable.

Question Are the math formulas provided?

Answer If a problem required a formula(s), then they should be provided in the question.

General Comments

The computer exam is a positive, convenient way to take the exam. The Pearson VUE people were friendly and helpful. The cubicles are quiet and well-lit, and the chairs are relatively comfortable. There is adequate table space and the computer was user friendly and non-threatening.

Conditions may vary considerably between testing locations. Please contact authors at 417-724-8348 or Email info@spansafetyworkshops.com. Feedback is greatly appreciated.

A listing of Pearson VUE center locations is available through the Pearson VUE website. More complete information can be obtained by calling or faxing the Board of Certified Safety Professionals. **Good Luck on the exam!**

Applied Study & Exam Techniques

The examination blueprint outlines how the items on an examination are distributed across domains and tasks/topics. Some keys to success include:

1. Analyzing knowledge gaps and identify strengths and weaknesses
2. Designing a solid examination study plan
3. Developing test-taking strategies

Converting your subject strengths and weaknesses into a study plan is likely to increase your overall examination score. Scoring well in one subject area can compensate for a weaker score in another subject area. However, there may not be enough items in your strong areas to achieve a passing score.
Note that knowledge and understanding are essential in passing the examination. Relying only on simulated examination items is not the best way to increase knowledge and understanding. Use simulated items to provide insight into the areas in which you should engage in additional study.

Knowing how to take the examination will help improve your score. The examination uses multiple-choice items with only one correct answer and three incorrect answers. Remember, the goal is to get as many items correct as possible. There is no penalty for selecting an incorrect answer. However, only correct answers count toward reaching the passing score.

- Read the items carefully.
    - Psychometricians design multiple choice questions so that all the possible answer choices are plausible. Use deductive and inductive reasoning to eliminate detractor answer choices.
- Understand the problem.
    - Consider the context
    - What is given? What is wanted?
- Use examination time wisely.
    - Conduct multiple passes solving the "easy" problems first and saving the challenging problems for the end.
- Complete all items.
    - Blank answers are scored as wrong answers.

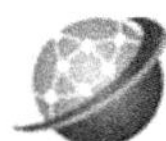

While studying resources, identify main thoughts or themes in the literature review. Draw on your experience and on professional and study references and rewrite important ideas in your own words. This helps you remember the concepts in context. Additional references are listed later in the workbook.

In establishing a good study regiment, it is important to find a place conducive to studying. A good study area should meet the following criteria:

- The study place should be chosen exclusively for the purpose of studying. Avoid using a garage, workshop, family room or other area that represents recreation or other distractions. Find a location that represents a study island, where study is the **only** activity.
- Selected study area should have good lighting, ventilation, be temperature controlled, comfortable and quiet.
- A large table or desk to spread necessary readily available study and reference materials is a must. The purpose is to dedicate a comfortable, personal space with minimal interruptions.

Securing a good place to study should eliminate as many external distractions as possible. Also, candidates should consider how to minimize internal distractions. Total elimination of external distractions is often possible; however, total elimination of internal distractions is nearly impossible and can only be minimized through focused thought.

Helpful hints for focusing the mind for studying include the following:

1. Set realistic time limits, determining what to study and keeping with a schedule. Studying a subject too long at one time can lead to daydreaming which reduces study effectiveness.
2. Personal factors can be distracters and result in additional frustration. All efforts should be attempted in avoiding personal issues. Rescheduling the SMS test date may be a consideration if serious personal problems exist.
3. Minimize dealing with outside details. Having too many obligations and/or responsibilities enables "brain creep". Consider keeping a notebook in the study area and jotting down appointments and details of projects as these brainstorms appear. It's impossible to totally prevent these details from surfacing, but by documenting them, it may free the mind to resume studies.

4. Being physically and mentally prepared to study is beneficial. Much of the following suggestions are common sense, but probably deserve repeating.
    - Eat a well-balanced diet. Increase protein intake; a proper level of blood sugar enhances studying effectiveness.
    - Get plenty of sleep. Establish and maintain a regular work/rest cycle.
    - Exercise is beneficial for more than just an exam preparation. Consider choosing a form of exercise that provides enjoyment and relaxation.
    - Avoid mental fatigue. Allocate down time for breaks. The average professional should study for the CSP exam for two to four weeks. DO NOT attempt to cram overnight.

The SPAN™ workbooks apply a Question & Answer format that allows candidates to concentrate on knowledge gaps and avoid over studying material in areas where the candidate already possess enough knowledge to pass the exam.

The research has been completed by the authors that have taken the exam and researched the blueprint areas of interest, developing targeted learning outcomes. This allows candidates to determine if their current level knowledge is adequate, or if a more in-depth understanding is required.

Fundamental to this technique is a good core of questions. The technique is intended to be useful to practitioners who have mastered the skills and tasks necessary to perform in the safety and health arena.

Most adult learners enjoy the process of learning. The difference lies in the ability to retain what is important to the accomplishment of a goal and reject what is not important. Embrace the aspect of professional development while preparing for the SMS examination.

When utilizing this workbook properly, the authors believe candidates can master those areas necessary to achieve the goal of passing the SMS examination with minimum effort on research and actual study. The technique also has some very beneficial side effects. Candidates will also find that the learning process will enhance skill sets in becoming an improved and more proficient safety and health practitioner.

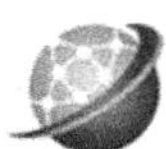

However, the process assumes candidates have the discipline to do the research and study the material where deficiencies may exist. Attempting to study using only the material presented in this workbook, becomes a risk for not being adequately prepared for the examination.

The steps to using the Q & A method:

1. Dead reckoning: using existing knowledge, experience, and test taking strategies, attempts to answer the question.

2. Process check: reviews the results of each practice session, and then studies the explanation.

3. Validate knowledge: was this a known or an unknown concept? Is the answer achieved with current knowledge base or the correct answer achieved by an educated guess or dumb luck?

Note: This is a critical step in the Q&A learning process and determines if one can proceed or needs to gain more knowledge on the subject. Additionally, is the knowledge base on this subject broad enough to answer questions of similar difficulty on the subject? *"True genius is an uncluttered mind armed with only relevant knowledge"(John R. Monteith).*

4. Filter: either move on or take notes. When comfortable with knowledge on the subject move on to the next question. However, if the current level of knowledge on the subject or other aspects of the subject feels inadequate, then take additional notes about the information that is needed.

5. Enhance deficiencies: Research and study deficient knowledge areas. After completing a set of questions and writing notes on information to study, a knowledge deficiency study plan can be developed. Then research and study the material necessary to enhance the required knowledge. The authors advise focusing on notes in the workbook and staying on subject. It is very easy to wander onto some other interesting subject and lose sight of the desired learning outcome. Keep the goal in mind to pass the test the first time!

A look at a representative question, answer and explanation will tend to illustrate and explain the process.

The concept of management review of an Occupational Health and Safety Management System (OHSMS) is to assure the SMS is suitable for the organization's needs, is adequately staffed and resourced, and is:
Effective at achieving desired results.
On schedule to meet implementation deadlines.
On track to meet financial goals.
Is clearly understood by all participants.

The correct answer is A because:
Top management must perform periodic management reviews of the OHSMS to ensure its continuing:

- Suitability (Does the system address conformance and meet the organization's needs?)
- Adequacy (Are the resources sufficient to maintain and improve the OHSMS?)
- Effectiveness (Is the system getting results?)

How much will candidates need to know about the subject of OHSMS? That is a key question an exam candidate should be asking right now. If OHSMS represents a strong area, a candidate probably has significant knowledge about the concepts outlined in references such as ANSI Z-10, ISO 45001, BSI 18001, OSHA VPP, and is comfortable with this question and the general subject. Another possibility is that one is basically knowledgeable on the subject but could use some more focused descriptors. Another scenario may be that a candidate knows very little about OHSMS, requiring more focus on concept details and application techniques.

How far into the topic does a student need to explore? The level of detail in the example question may serve as a representative indicator. Beyond the basics, another key indicator is the repetition of the workbook question. Content frequently appearing with only minor changes in question format indicates that the subject matter is important, and authors anticipate the actual exam will have several questions dealing with that subject.

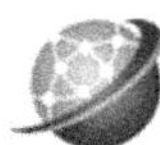

The Q & A method of studying is a proven method. The basic outline is delivered with questions and students can then determine individual levels of subject knowledge. When additional knowledge is required, they can conduct more research and study to develop the required knowledge or skill. This learning technique has proven to be successful for many different levels of adult learners because **the individual** determines what material to study.

Again, please contact the authors at info@spansafetyworkshops.com with any questions or feedback on these study materials.

Key Consensus, Voluntary, Guidance Standards:

- ANSI-ASSE Z10- Occupational Health & Safety Management Systems
- ANSI ASSE Z490- Practices and Criteria for Safety & Health Training
- ANSI/ASSE Z590.2-2003 – Criteria for Establishing the Scope and Functions of the Professional Safety Position
- ANSI/ Z590.3-2011 – Prevention Through Design
- BSI 18001-Safety & Health Managements systems
- ISO 14000 Environmental Managements Systems
- ISO 31000 Risk Management Principles
- ISO 30010 Risk Management Assessment Techniques
- ISO 19011 Auditing Management Systems
- NFPA 10 Fire Extinguishers
- NFPA 13 Sprinkler Systems
- NFPA 30 Flammable Liquids
- NFPA 70E Electrical
- NFPA 101 Life Safety Code

Domain 1: Management Systems

Domain 1: Management Systems 20%
Knowledge of: 1. Principles and common elements of safety management systems (e.g., continuous improvement, safety processes, controls, measurement, standards, implementation) 2. Principles and techniques for encouraging employee involvement and commitment (e.g., value-based safety) 3. Principles and techniques for encouraging management commitment to safety (e.g., voluntary protection program (VPP), mission statement, management involvement in jobsite assessment) 4. Techniques and principles for goal setting (e.g., SMART) 5. Principles and techniques of internal audits 6. Competency/skills assessment management systems (e.g., new hire orientation, assurance of experience, job skills, on the job training) as it pertains to worker safety 7. General concepts of effective trainings (e.g., learning retention, adult learning principles, training delivery) 8. Recordkeeping related to training and education (e.g., annual, one-time, recertification or retraining) 9. Management of corrective actions (e.g., follow up, follow through, closure of actions, time periods, tracking corrective actions) 10. Unsafe conditions and acts and how they relate to incidents (e.g., Swiss cheese model, bowtie model) 11. Management of change (MOC) procedure and organizational change process 12. Common elements of contractor or multi-employer worksite safety programs (e.g., prequalification, selecting, monitoring, managing risk between contractor and host)
Skill to: 1. Recognize leading and lagging indicators 2. Set and prioritize safety-related goals 3. Assess training needs (regulatory and risk-based)

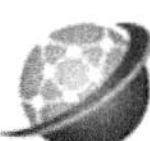

Occupational Health and Safety Management Systems

A management system is a set of interrelated elements used to establish policy and objectives and implement strategies to achieve those objectives. A management system includes organizational structure, planning activities, responsibilities, practices, procedures, processes, and resources. The conventional model for a management framework that follows a logical progression of activities aimed at improving the performance of the organization is the "Plan, Do, Check, Act" or PDCA cycle.

An organization may choose to implement a management system for many reasons, such as enhancing business performance through the following:

- Developing a management structure that is effective and responsive to the organization's needs
- Making operational improvements
- Changing the operational culture
- Marketing opportunities and improving public image
- Improving relationships with regulators
- Enhancing the ability to meet regulatory requirements and reduced costs from penalties
- Providing for greater employee involvement, awareness and commitment to performance, and improving morale
- Complying with a client's requirements

Occupational Health & Safety Management Systems (OHSMS's) consist of six "core elements". Each core element is important and necessary to ensure the success of the overall system. All the elements are interrelated and interdependent. The core elements are:

1) **Management Leadership:** Managers at all levels of the organization demonstrate their commitment to improved safety and health, communicate their commitment, and document performance. Managers make safety and health a top priority, establish goals and objectives, provide adequate resources and support, and set a good example.

Management Leadership
• Establish clear safety and health objectives for the OHSMS and operationally define the actions needed to achieve those objectives.
• Designate one or more individuals with overall responsibility for implementing and maintaining the OHSMS.
• Provide sufficient resources to ensure effective OHSMS implementation.

Employee Participation: Management actively involves employees in all aspects of the OHSMS—setting goals, identifying and reporting hazards, investigating incidents, tracking progress, among others. All employees understand their roles and responsibilities under the OHSMS and what they need to do to carry them out effectively. Employees are encouraged to communicate openly with management and report safety and health concerns. Any barriers to participation (for example, language or other) are addressed.

Employee [Worker] Participation
• Consult with employees in developing and implementing the system and involve them in updating and evaluating the OHSMS.
• Include employees in workplace inspections, incident investigations, and solutions.
• Encourage employees to report concerns, such as hazards, injuries, illnesses and near misses.

Hazard Identification and Assessment: Processes and procedures are put in place to continually identify workplace hazards and evaluate risks. An initial assessment of existing hazards and control measures is followed by periodic reassessments to identify new hazards and monitor the effectiveness of prevention and control measures.

Hazard Identification and Risk Assessment
• Identify, assess and document workplace hazards with activities such as soliciting input from workers, inspecting the workplace and reviewing available information on hazards and risks.
• Investigate incidents that in involve both injuries and illnesses and near misses to identify hazards that may have caused them. The purpose is prevention.
• Inform employees of the hazards and risks in the workplace.

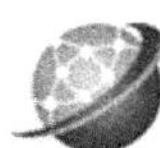

Hazard Prevention and Control: Processes, procedures, and programs are created and implemented to eliminate or control workplace hazards and achieve safety and health goals and objectives. Progress in implementing controls is tracked.

Hazard Prevention and Control
• Establish and implement a plan to prioritize and control hazards and risks identified in the workplace.
• Provide both interim and permanent controls that reduce the risk of exposure to hazards and protect employees.
• Verify that all control measures are implemented and are effective.
• Discuss the hazard control plan with affected employees.

Education and Training: All employees are trained to carry out their responsibilities under the SHMS. In addition, all employees are trained to recognize workplace hazards and protect themselves and their coworkers from these hazards.

Education and Training
• Provide education and training to employees in a language and vocabulary they can understand to ensure that they know: o Procedures for reporting injuries, illnesses and safety and health concerns. o How to recognize hazards. o Ways to eliminate, control or reduce hazards. o Elements of the program. o How to participate in the program.
• Conduct refresher education and training programs periodically.

System Evaluation and Improvement: Progress and performance effectiveness of control measures are periodically evaluated. Processes are established to monitor OHSMS performance, verify implementation, identify deficiencies and opportunities for improvement, and take necessary actions to improve the SHMS and overall safety and health performance.

System Evaluation and Continuous Improvement
• Conduct a periodic review of the safety management system to determine if it has been implemented as designed and is making progress towards achieving its goals.
• Modify the program, as necessary, to correct deficiencies.
• Continuously look for ways to improve the OHSMS.

Management Leadership

An effective Occupational Safety and Health Management System (OHSMS) requires leadership and commitment from top management. Management leadership provides the motivating force and the resources for organizing and controlling activities within an organization. In an effective OHSMS holds worker safety and health as a fundamental value of the organization. Ideally, this means that concern for every aspect of the safety and health of all workers throughout the job site is demonstrated.

Effective OHSMS leadership:

- Creates safety and health management system policy and procedures.
- Establishes and communicates organizational goals and the pathways (objectives) to achieve goals
- Demonstrates visible management involvement
- Assigns and communicating responsibility, authority and resources to responsible parties and holding those parties accountable.
- Encourages employees to report hazards, symptoms, injuries and illnesses, and identify programs or policies which discourage this reporting.

Successful top managers, superintendents, and supervisors use a variety of techniques that visibly involve them in the safety and health protection of their workers. Managers and supervisors should look for methods that fit their style and workplace conditions.

Examples of visible safety leadership:

- Getting out where you can be seen, informally or through formal inspections.
- Being accessible by incorporating safety and health into operational conversations and standard operating procedures.
- Promptly reward acceptable safety performance and correct at risk situations.
- Leading by example, by knowing and following the rules employees are expected to follow.
- Active involvement by participating in the workplace safety and health solutions.

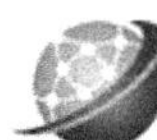

Ten Principles of Safety Management[21]

1).	An unsafe act, an unsafe condition, and an accident are all symptoms management systems problems.
2).	Circumstances that will produce severe injuries are predictable and can be identified and controlled.
3).	Safety should be managed like any other company function. Management should direct the safety effort by setting achievable goals and by planning, organizing, and controlling to achieve them.
4).	The key to effective line safety performance is management procedures that fix accountability.
5).	The function of safety is to locate and define the operational errors that allow accidents to occur. This function can be carried out in two ways: A) by asking why accidents happen - searching for their root causes B) by asking whether certain known effective controls are being utilized
6).	The causes of unsafe behavior can be identified and classified. Some of the classifications are Overload (the improper matching of a person's capacity with the load); Traps, and the worker's decision to error. Each cause is one which can be controlled.
7).	In most cases, unsafe behavior is normal human behavior; it is the result of normal people reacting to their environment. Management's job is to change the environment that leads to unsafe behavior.
8).	There are three major subsystems that must be dealt with in building an effective safety system: the physical; the managerial; the behavioral
9).	The safety system should fit the culture of the organization.
10).	There is no one right way to achieve safety in an organization; however, for a safety system to be effective, the system must: Force supervisory performance; involve middle management; Have top management visibly showing their commitment; Have employee participation; be flexible; be perceived as positive.

[21] Adapted from Dan Peterson, 2003.

Employee Participation

Employee involvement provides the means through which workers develop and express their own commitment to safety and health, for both themselves and their fellow workers. It is also key to getting accurate risk assessments, workers closest to the operations usually have the best knowledge of the methods, tasks, breakdowns and problems. The findings and lessons arising from all evaluation and corrective action activities become part of the information that feeds back to the employee participation process

Employees should be involved because:

- They are the persons most in contact with potential safety and health hazards. They have a vested interest in effective protection systems.
- Group decisions have the advantage of the group's wider range of experience.
- Employees are more likely to support and use programs in which they have input.
- Employees who are encouraged to offer their ideas and whose contributions are taken seriously are more satisfied and productive on the job.

Examples of employee participation include:
Participating on joint labor-management committees and other advisory or specific purpose committees.

- Conducting site inspections.
- Analyzing routine hazards in each step of a job or process and preparing safe work practices or controls to eliminate or reduce exposure.
- Developing and revising the site safety and health rules.
- Training both current and newly hired employees.
- Providing programs and presentations at safety and health meetings.
- Conducting accident/incident investigations.
- Reporting hazards.
- Fixing hazards within your control.
- Supporting your fellow workers by providing feedback on risks and assisting them in eliminating hazards.
- Participating in accident/incident investigations.
- Performing a pre-use or change analysis for new equipment or processes to identify hazards up front before use.

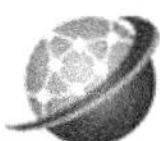

Education and Training

Education and training are critical for developing the skills and knowledge of workplace hazards and how employees protect themselves from those hazards. It is important that everyone in the workplace is properly trained. This includes the worker to the supervisors, managers, contractors, and part-time and temporary workers. It is important to distinguish that training is not education. Education is generally measured by tenure: you spent a day in the seminar or four years in college. Training, on the other hand, is measured by what you can do when you've completed it.

- Training delivers the skills to do something rather than just know about something. Training involves practical application of the knowledge and skill.

- Education is all about learning the theory and more importantly, transferring that learning into new or different situations. Traditionally, an education may reinforce knowledge in which that you already have a foundation.

Supervisors and managers should be trained to recognize hazards and understand their responsibilities. The organization should establish a process to:

- Define and assess the OHSMS competence needed for employees and contractors
- Ensure through appropriate education, training, or other methods that employees and contractors are aware of applicable OHSM requirements and competent in their responsibilities.
- Ensure effective access to education and training and remove barriers to participation.
- Ensure training is provided in a language trainees understand.
- Ensure training is ongoing and timely.
- Ensure trainers are competent to train employees.

Training can help to develop the knowledge and skills needed to understand workplace hazards and safe procedures. It is most effective when integrated into a company's overall training in performance requirements and job practices.

The content of a company's training program and the methods of presentation should reflect the needs and characteristics of the workforce. Therefore, identification of needs is an important early step in training design. Involving everyone in this process and in the subsequent teaching can be highly effective.

These principles of training should be followed to maximize effectiveness:

- Training needs assessment, will training solve the issue.
- Measurable learning [performance] objectives.
- Trainees should understand the purpose of the training.
- Information should be organized to maximize effectiveness.
- People learn best when they can immediately practice and apply newly acquired knowledge and skills.
- As trainees practice, they should get feedback.
- People learn in different ways, so effective training will incorporate a variety of training methods.

Some examples of health and safety training needed:

- Orientation training for new hires, site workers and contractors
- JSAs, SOPs, and other hazard recognition training
- Training required by OSHA standards: hazard communication, fall protection, operator, electrical, PPE, etc.
- Hazard identification, control and reporting
- Safety inspections
- Accident investigation training
- Emergency drills

Managers and supervisors should also be included in the training plan. Training for managers should emphasize the importance of their role in visibly supporting the safety and health program and setting a good example. Supervisors should receive training in company policies and procedures, as well as hazard detection and control, accident investigation, handling of emergencies, and how to train and reinforce training.

The entire workforce needs periodic refresher training to reinforce OHSMS goals and objectives.

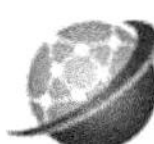

Plan to evaluate the training program when initially designing the training. If the evaluation is done right, it can identify your program's strengths and weaknesses, and provide a basis for future program changes.

Keeping training records will help ensure that everyone who should get training does. Training documentation may include:

- The targeted audience and learning objective(s)
- Sources used to develop training materials
- Training evaluation methods
- The date location and duration of the training
- Name and description of the course
- Names of trainers delivering the training
- The delivery materials used
- The trainees participating in the training
- The trainees' successful completion of the training
- Certification of training and testing

Domain 1 Quiz 1 Questions

1) If an organization's occupational health and safety management system is to succeed, as described in *ANSI/ASSE* Z10, there are two critical components, top management leadership and
   A) Supervisor accountability.
   B) Employee participation.
   C) OHS written policy.
   D) Sustainable safety observation program.

2) Auditing conformance with ISO 14001 and OHSAS 18001 management systems is important for companies. Which of the following best provides minimally suitable verification that the company is reviewing proposed or new legal requirements as they apply to the organization?
   A) A document identifying the date of any review of new or proposed legal requirements and a statement determining applicability.
   B) A certified letter from the legal department stating that the company complies with all legal requirements.
   C) An electronic message from a legal update review service, signifying that new legal requirements are routinely conveyed to the company.
   D) A signed report outlining legal requirements applicable to the organization.

3) British Standard OHSAS 18001, states that a successful management system should be based on all the following **except**
   A) A generic occupational health and safety policy.
   B) Identification of occupational health and safety risks and legal requirements.
   C) Objectives, targets, and programs that guarantee continuing improvement.
   D) Management activities that manage occupational health and safety risks.

4) To ensure the safety and health of employees, an employer must:
   A) Maintain the workplace in a cost-effective way.
   B) Ensure that external fire doors are held open always.
   C) Maintain the workplace in a safe condition.
   D) Ensure that fire doors are kept locked.

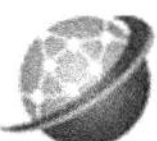

5) The **primary** purpose of ISO 19011 is to provide guidance on
   A) Designing and developing S&H systems.
   B) Improving environmental control systems.
   C) Implementation of an SH&E management system.
   D) Managing and conducting quality and environmental management system audits.

6) Which of the following is the **least important** purpose of an Occupational Health and Safety system audit?
   A) Gather data for management performance reports and assure appropriate barriers are in place for worker participation.
   B) Determine and document compliance and conformance status.
   C) Develop a basis for optimizing and allocating resources.
   D) Improve OHSMS performance and implement risk management program.

7) Which **best** describes how to implement specific and consistent operational tasks for how to do a job safely?
   A) Regulation.
   B) Safety Manual.
   C) Policy.
   D) Procedure.

8) One key to success when implementing a safety change initiative in a global organization is:
   A) Frequent audits to assure conformance with corporate policies and procedures.
   B) Document all conversations in case of disputes during the implementation.
   C) Focus more on outcomes and less on processes used to achieve them.
   D) Embed senior corporate managers in all foreign facilities.

9) To effectively oversee a safety & health management system, safety directors should ________ as many levels of management as possible.
   A) Report to.
   B) Acquire access to.
   C) Cite violations of standards to.
   D) Have budgets approved by.

10) All of the following are included in ANSI/ASSE Z10 **except**
   A) S&H policy development.
   B) Employee participation.
   C) Management review.
   D) Evaluation and corrective action.

11) Which of the following is the **least** accurate description of change analysis?
   A) Change analysis in safety should reflect the multiple succession realities rather than rely on possibly one-dimensional detection-correction of a single contributory change.
   B) If a system has been operating in a stable manner but is now experiencing difficulties, change is probably not the basis of the problem.
   C) Sensitivity to approaching or plausible change is a key component in the work of a good, experienced manager or safety professional.
   D) In multifaceted systems, consideration must be given to accumulation of change, for example adjustments made two years ago combined with a modification made a month ago may produce the undesired event.

12) When ANSI standards are developed or revised, what must be identified?
   A) The stakeholders that are impacted by the standard.
   B) The cost of implementation on the stakeholders.
   C) The impact of the environmental life cycle.
   D) The regulatory requirements for compliance with the standard.

13) In project management, work that must be performed to deliver a product, service or result with the specified features and functions is called the:
   A) Project schedule.
   B) Project scope.
   C) Project scope statement.
   D) Project scope management plan.

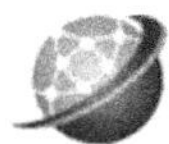

14) A new Safety Director was hired by a company that traditionally has had a "paper safety program". The director has a staff of three and reports to one of three vice presidents. The rates for the company are much higher than the industrial average. The initial assessment is that there is very little interest in safety at any level. The Safety Director has been given authority to increase the safety staff and has been given a sizable increase in department budget. After having hired new staff and reorganizing the department, the next step should be to:

A) Increase the safety training effort for all employees.
B) Organize a safety committee and get management to appoint members.
C) Start an inspection program to identify areas that need attention.
D) Integrate safety accountability into job descriptions, appraisals, and objectives.

15) Recently, numerous tools have been left behind after maintenance has been completed. What is the **best** way to increase tool accountability and improve or eliminate the problem?

A) Associate employee number to tool usage.
B) Develop a remotely monitored system.
C) Implement an automated bar-coding system.
D) Install a computerized system.

16) According to ANSI Z10, organizational goals and objectives should meet targets that are:

A) Measurable, actionable, rigorous, specific, open ended
B) Special, measurable, actionable, opportunistic, timed
C) Specific, measurable, actionable, realistic, time-bound
D) Subjective, actionable, regulatory, measureable, time-bound

17) Which ISO standard series covers environmental management?

A) 9001
B) 19011
C) 31001
D) 14001

18) The steps for the continuous improvement safety process are the same as in the continuous quality improvement process. These include all of the following **except:**
   A) Specify standards.
   B) Measure compliance.
   C) Track procedures.
   D) Provide feedback on improvement.

19) The traditional three E's of safety management represented engineering, education and enforcement. A modern conept for worker participation replaces enforcement with:
   A) Encouragement.
   B) Exemption.
   C) Entitlement.
   D) Empowerment.

20) An accident causation model that represents a layered approach to safety and security is called:
   A) Swiss Cheese.
   B) Bow tie.
   C) 5-whys.
   D) Job Safety Analysis.

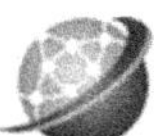

Domain 1 Quiz 1 Answers

1) Answer B:
   According to *ANSI/ASSE Z10*, top management leadership and employee participation are the main divisions in the scope of this standard.

2) Answer A:
   A member of the management team must certify that such reviews were conducted and must include date of review and findings of applicability. This type of written certification is common practice in auditing methods because it is not practical for auditors to observe and verify that **all** management processes were conducted.

3) Answer A:
   OHSAS 18001 is an *Occupation Health and Safety Assessment Series* for health and safety management systems. It is intended to help an organization to control occupational health and safety risks. It was developed in response to widespread demand for a recognized standard against which to be certified and assessed. OHSAS 18001 will measure a company's managements system regarding several dimensions. The extent of application will depend on such factors as the occupational health and safety policy of the organization, the nature of its activities, and conditions under which it operates. A successful management system should be based on the following**:**

   - An occupational health and safety policy appropriate for the company.
   - Identification of occupational health and safety risks and legal requirements.
   - Objectives, targets, and programs that ensure continual improvements.
   - Management activities that control the occupational health and safety risks.
   - Monitoring of the occupational health and safety system performance.
   - Continual reviews, evaluation, and system improvement.

4) Answer C:
According to ANSI/ASSE/IEC/ISO 31010 (Z690.3-2011) Risk Assessment Techniques National Adoption of: IEC/ISO 31010:2009
The purpose of risk assessment is to provide evidence-based information and analysis to make informed decisions on how to treat risks and how to select between options. Some of the principal benefits of performing risk assessment include:
- understanding the risk and its potential impact upon objectives;
- providing information for decision makers; contributing to the understanding of risks, to assist in selection of treatment options;
- identifying the important contributors to risks and weak links in systems and organizations;
- comparing of risks in alternative systems, technologies or approaches;
- communicating risks and uncertainties;
- assisting with establishing priorities;
- contributing towards incident prevention based upon post incident investigation;
- selecting different forms of risk treatment;
- meeting regulatory requirements;
- providing information that will help evaluate whether the risk should be accepted when compared with pre-defined criteria;
- assessing risks for end-of-life disposal

These processes are what keeps the employees and workplace safe.

5) Answer D:
ISO 19011 is an international standard that sets forth guidelines for:
- quality management systems auditing
- environmental management systems auditing

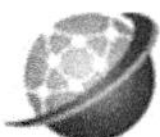

6) Answer A:
OHSMS audits are performed for the following reasons (listed in order of importance):
1) determine and document compliance and conformance status
2) improve overall OHSM system performance
3) evaluate implementation organizational risk management decisions
4) increase the overall level of OHSMS awareness and participation
5) continuous improvement of risk management control systems
6) demonstrate management leadership through "walking the talk"
7) protect company from potential liabilities
8) develop a basis for optimizing OHSMS resources
9) assess achievement of OHSMS goals and objectives

7) Answer D:
According to definitions in the ISO 45001 standard:

- **Policy** represents the intentions and direction of an *organization* (3.1), as formally expressed by its *top management* (3.12).
- **Process** (3.25) is the set of interrelated or interacting activities which transforms inputs into outputs. This constitutes one of the common terms and core definitions for ISO management system standards given in Annex SL of the Consolidated ISO Supplement to the ISO/IEC Directives.
- **Procedure** is a specified way to carry out an activity or a *process* (3.25)

The OHSAS 18001 specification requires only minimal documentation. It is important that documented OH&S procedures are developed and adequately controlled. A compilation of documents that form the basis for the management system is normally involve overall policies and specific procedures to be following to implement the Occupational Safety and Health Management System (OHSMS). According to author Joe Kausek of OHSAS 18001 *Designing and Implementing an Effective Health and Safety Management System*, clause 4.4.4 requires electronic or hard copy of the information that provides an overall description of the main elements of the OHSMS, how these elements interact and reference to any documents that describe these activities in more detail. Normally, the first step in establishing control is to develop a master listing of the policies, procedures, instructions, forms, and other documents that form the basis for the management system. This is normally called the Master List.

8) Answer C:

Implementing a safety change initiative in a global organization can be difficult because of how different cultures view safety and risk management. It is important to incorporate cultural elements into the management system. (Global Solutions, Inc. 2011). A successful strategy for assessing the management of risk at local in-country facilities is to:

- Focus on outcomes: What is the risk?
- How is it managed? Is the risk adequately controlled?
- Allow for cultural, technological, legal, regulatory, health care, social system, and other differences in developing solutions to risk control challenges, findings, and other implementation strategies. The best advice:
- Ask a lot of questions before mandating risk-control solutions for your global facilities

9) Answer B:

Access to managers throughout an organization will assist the safety director in developing an accepted, consistent, effective safety management system. It is critical that top management understand and support the safety & health management system. If the safety function reports at a high level in a company that does not value safety, the level of reporting is irrelevant.

10) Answer A:

ANSI/ASSE Z10 provides the blueprint for widespread benefits in health and safety, as well as in productivity, financial, performance, quality, and other organizational and business objectives. The seven sections include Management Leadership and Employee Participation, Planning, Implementation and Operation, Evaluation and Corrective Action, Management Review.

11) Answer B:

In William G. Johnson's book *MORT Safety Assurance Systems*, he states that "change is the mother of trouble", referencing the following areas of concern:

- Change analysis in safety should reflect the multiple sequence realities rather than rely on possibly simplistic detection-correction of a single causative change.
- If a system has been operating in a stable manner but now experiencing difficulties, change is probably the cause of the problem.
- Sensitivity to impending or probable change is a key component in the

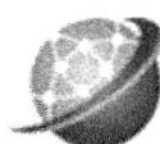

work of a good, experienced manage or safety professional.

- In complex systems, attention must be given to compounding of change. For example, a change made two years ago combined with a change made a month ago may produce the undesired event.

12) Answer A:

According to ANSI Essential Requirements: Due process requirements for American National Standards protocols section 2.5.1 Project Initiation Notification (PINS); At the initiation of a project to develop or revise an American National Standard, notification shall be transmitted to ANSI using the Project Initiation Notification System (PINS) form, or its equivalent, for announcement in *Standards Action*. A statement shall be submitted and published as part of the PINS announcement that shall include:

- an explanation of the need for the project, including, if it is the case, a statement of intent to submit the standard for consideration as an ISO, IEC or ISO/IEC JTC-1 standard; and
- Identification of the stakeholders (e.g., telecom, consumer, medical, environmental, etc.) likely to be directly impacted by the standard.

13) Answer B:

This is the definition of a **project scope** which includes the specific scope of work objectives. Plan safety through the project life cycle to consider work activities, hazards, risk, multi-employer worksite issues. The **work breakdown structure (WBS)** organizes and defines the total scope of the project. Each descending level represents an increasingly detailed definition of project work. The WBS is decomposed into work packages. The deliverable orientation of the hierarchy includes both internal and external deliverables.

14) Answer D:

According to Dr. Roger l. Brauer in *Safety and Health for Engineers*, making safety part of a supervisor's or manager's daily responsibilities and including it in their appraisals, job descriptions, and applying it to possible promotions and salary increases is the primary requirement for a successful safety program. When determining the staffing level at given locations, areas to consider are the injury rate, the number of recognized hazards and the worker compensation costs per employee. The number of employees will impact the final decision but is not as important as the previous three considerations.

15) Answer C:

The bar-coding system would be the best choice for tool accountability. In this type of system, tools entering an area would be scanned prior to an employee entering. When work was completed, tools would be scanned as employee left the area. If a tool were left inside, the final scan list would show that a tool had entered and was not scanned as having left the area. This type of system is widely used in industries where an errant tool left in an area could cause damage or result in other severe consequences. Associating employee numbers to tools checked out from a tool crib would aid in accounting for who was using certain tools. However, just checking out the tool would not be sufficient for accounting as to the location of the tool (i.e.; tool bag, left behind).

16) Answer C:

Objectives should meet targets, ANSI Z-10 using the example of "SMART" criteria:

- Specific—Clearly defined desired outcome
- Measurable—Concrete metric for success
- Actionable—Written as a concrete action plan
- Realistic—Practical in its scope
- Time-bounded—A specific timeframe is set

When choosing an appropriate organizational model, a manager should understand that there are multiple arrangements that will produce the best result with minimum difficulty when the organization operates. Given individual discretion and the fact that some configurations appear to influence employee performance and satisfaction, managers should consider carefully the behavioral implications when making decisions.

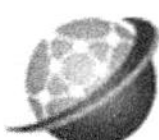

17) Answer D:
The ISO 9000 (“quality management”) and ISO 14000 ("environmental management") families are among ISO's most widely known standards in safety. ISO 9000 has become an international reference for quality requirements in business to business dealings, and ISO 14000 looks set to achieve at least as much, if not more, in helping organizations to meet their environmental challenges. The **ISO 9000** family addresses **"quality management"**. This means what the organization does to fulfill:

- customer's quality requirements
- applicable regulatory requirements, while aiming to enhance customer satisfaction
- continual improvement of performance in pursuit of these objectives

The **ISO 14000** family addresses **"environmental management"**. This means what the organization does to

- minimize harmful effects on environment caused by its activities
- achieve continual improvement of its environmental performance

18) Answer C:
Most of the Behavior Based Safety experts define the “continuous improvement safety process as consisting of

- specifying standards
- measuring compliance
- providing feedback on improvements

19) Answer D:
Modern safety management theory embraces a “people-based or value-driven” approach to safety. Substituting concepts of empowerment, ownership, and interpersonal trust for more traditional safety terms such as compliance and enforcement.

20) Answer A:
The **Swiss cheese model** of accident causation is a **model** used in risk analysis and risk management, including aviation safety, engineering, healthcare, emergency service organizations, and as the principle behind layered security, as used in computer security and defense in depth. It likens human systems to multiple slices of Swiss cheese, stacked side by side, in which the risk of a threat becoming a reality is mitigated by the differing layers and types of defenses which are "layered" behind each other. Therefore, in theory, lapses and

weaknesses in one defense do not allow a risk to materialize, since other defenses also exist, to prevent a single point of weakness. A **BowTie** is a diagram that visualizes the risk you are dealing with in just one, easy to understand picture. The diagram is shaped like a bow-tie, creating a clear differentiation between proactive and reactive risk management. The power of a BowTie diagram is that it gives you an overview of multiple plausible scenarios, in a single picture. In short, it provides a simple, visual explanation of a risk that would be much more difficult to explain otherwise.

5 Whys is an iterative interrogative technique used to explore the cause-and-effect relationships underlying a particular problem. The primary goal of the technique is to determine the root cause of a defect or problem by repeating the question "Why?"

A **job safety analysis** (JSA) is a procedure which helps integrate accepted safety and health principles and practices into a task or job operation. In a JSA, each basic step of the job is to identify potential hazards and to recommend the safest way to do the job

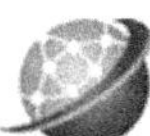

Domain 1 Quiz 2 Questions

1) At minimum, documentation of training includes student name, topic outline, objectives, date and:
   A) Instructor name and qualifications.
   B) Multi-media presentation.
   C) Pre-and post test scores.
   D) Literacy equivalency.

2) Which of the following is **least important** when performing a task analysis?
   A) Observing the task.
   B) Performing the task.
   C) Cost of retraining.
   D) Reviewing company written SOPs and policies.

3) When a supervisor is evaluating a subordinate during the annual employee performance report cycle, which factor is **most** important?
   A) Safety performance.
   B) Attentiveness to minutiae.
   C) Measurable objective criterion.
   D) Magnitude of production in comparison to peers.

4) Which of the following training methods is **primarily** used to find new, innovative approaches to issues?
   A) Meeting.
   B) Brainstorming.
   C) Case study.
   D) Role playing.

5) Enabling learning objectives should define measurable skills, knowledge, or behaviors required to achieve performance objectives. Which of the is the **least** measurable objective?
   A) The supervisor will understand how to be safe on the workplace.
   B) The worker will identify hazardous chemicals.
   C) The operator will troubleshoot a machine operating cycle.
   D) The employee will enter data into the work order system.

6) For training to be effective, training objectives should be established and measured. Which statement about training objectives is **least** effective on performance outcomes?
   A) Training objectives should be reasonable and practical.
   B) Training objectives must be measurable.
   C) Training objectives should be obtainable.
   D) Training objectives must be written.

7) A study that is a systematic analysis of an organization, or detailed job/task, to determine how training can help the organization to improve its safety, success or efficiency or if the specific job/task can be improved is called a:
   A) Managerial analysis.
   B) Training analysis.
   C) Needs analysis.
   D) Task analysis.

8) Which of the following would be of the **greatest** importance when defining training goals?
   A) Regulations.
   B) Worker interviews.
   C) Job task analysis.
   D) Critical incident analysis.

9) Learner reaction to instruction greatly impacted by facilitator behaviors. Which learner performance outcome is **least likely** to occur?
   A) Observers learn by watching and imitating others; they tend to behave as they have seen others behave.
   B) Observers will imitate a model who is passionate about his/her topic.
   C) Observers will imitate a model when they see the model being rewarded for his/her actions.
   D) Observers will imitate a model when they see the model being punished for his/her actions.

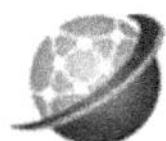

10) Learning objectives are brief, clear and concise statements of what the learner should be able to do as an outcome of training. All the following are completed prior to designing the learning objectives **except**:

A) The needs analysis should determine if training is the solution.
B) A task analysis and supervisor discussions will identify performance requirements.
C) Lesson plans should be implemented consistently to all affected workers.
D) Performance criteria is established and documented.

11) The **primary** considerations during development and evaluation of a training program for operating a new piece of equipment are

A) Management expectations, participant expectations, skills and knowledge.
B) A detailed course on the engineering of design specifications for equipment from the manufacturer.
C) Instructional strategies, participant expectations, and equipment safety signage.
D) Operationally bypass specific safe guards, minimize exposure to equipment hazards, and management expectations

12) A common safety training technique when facilitating work team learning is the case study. Which is **most** correct about the use of a case study as a learning strategy?

A) Case studies must always involve fictitious situations or incidents so that no one group, or individual will feel threatened.
B) Case studies should be written and distributed as handouts to be most effective since most tradecraft employees have short attention spans.
C) Case studies are good problem-solving tools and can be used effectively with brainstorming activities and group discussions.
D) Case studies involving real situations should only be used if they can be presented by the actual employees/responders involved in the situation or incident.

13) Adult learning theory has established universal assumptions of adult learner needs. Which statement is **least** likely considered when designing hazard awareness training?

A) Adults have experience and need to control their learning.
B) Adults need to know why learning information is relevant.
C) Adults need to be provided with written training materials to make meaning of learning content.
D) Adults need to know how to apply knowledge and skill for successful performance.

14) Safety and Health Management Systems such as BSI 18001 series and ANSI/ASSE Z10-2012 are built on established principles and process. Which of the following phases involves management verification in a systems process?

A) Plan.
B) Do.
C) Check.
D) Act.

15) Safety and health training can involve many diverse delivery schemes and training techniques. Often group methods are used to increase effectiveness of training and active involvement of participants. Which of the following would be the **best** use of the role playing?

A) For human relations training.
B) For job training in a one-on-one environment.
C) To exemplify the complexities of a step-by-step comprehensive industrial task.
D) For in-depth technical topics.

16) Which of the following is the **most** accurate concerning guided disccussion?

A) Individual understanding is not particularly important.
B) Not particularly appropriate for problem solving.
C) Success largely dependent upon the skills of the facilitator.
D) Success depends entirely on the amount of materials covered.

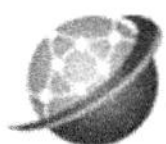

17) Which of the following is the **least** valuable quality of interactive computer-assisted training (sometimes called distance learning)?
   A) Works well for organizations with small workforces.
   B) Functions well for organizations that cannot remove large portions of the workforce from the job at one time.
   C) Permits instructors to interact with each other without restrictions.
   D) Trainees can engage in training at their own pace.

18) When selecting a communications medium for a training presentation, which features are listed in **increasing** order for learner retention?
   A) Experience, auditory, words.
   B) Words, visual pictures, experience.
   C) Displays, auditory, demonstrations.
   D) Demonstrations, auditory, words.

19) Selecting the media to be used for presenting instructional content:
   A) Requires only a knowledge of specific course objectives.
   B) Should be done only after a planning process that includes content analysis, audience analysis and other steps.
   C) Partly determine what content can be included and should precede content analysis.
   D) Is the first step in instructional design.

20) Safety trainers often attempt to change the way an audience views their procedures or actions. A **primary** way to help facilitate change is by
   A) Allowing everyone to express their point of view.
   B) Following lesson plan without interruptions.
   C) Allowing limited questions at end of presentation.
   D) Pointing out how change will affect the workplace.

Domain 1 Quiz 2 Answers

1) Answer A:

At minimum, documentation of training includes, student name, topic outline, objectives, date, instructor name and qualifications. Training records listing the dates courses were presented, the names of the individual course attendees, the names of those students successfully completing each course, and the number of training certificates issued to each successful student. Record retention policies may vary, based on regulations and company policy. Generally records should be maintained for a minimum of five years after the date of training.

According to ANSI Z490.1-2012, the written training program plan shall include procedures for document control. A record keeping system shall be established for controlling all records and documents required to ensure that:

- They are retrievable, readily identifiable, and maintained in an orderly manner.
- They are current, accurate, legible, and dated (including revision dates).
- They are retained for a specified period.
- They meet applicable legislative or regulatory requirements.

Development records shall identify:

- The target audience and stated learning objective(s).
- Sources used to develop training materials.
- The persons designing and developing the training and their qualifications.
- All training materials developed for the course.
- Plans for evaluation and continuous improvement of the course.

Delivery records for each training event shall identify:

- The date, location, and duration of the training.
- The name and description of the course.
- The names and qualifications of persons delivering the training.
- The delivery materials used.
- The trainees participating in the training.
- The trainees successfully completing the training.

Evaluation records shall be retained for:

- Training evaluation; and
- Periodic reevaluation of a course.

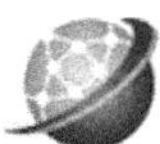

2) Answer C:

The cost of retraining is not a factor when conducting a task analysis. Task analysis is the process of detailing task performance. The task performance details should describe how the task is performed (performance steps), under what conditions it is performed, and how well the individual must perform it (performance standards).

Task analysis is the process of breaking a task down to identify the:

1. Component steps of a task.
2. Sequence of those steps.
3. Conditions under which the task will be performed.
4. Task cues.
5. Standard of performance that must be achieved, expressed in terms of accuracy, completeness, sequence, or speed.

A combination of the following methods and techniques can be used to identify the tasks and compile a ***task inventory***. More than one method should be used since each method has its inherent strengths and weaknesses.

- The content method of data collection is a review of all available literature.
- The interview/survey method involves interviewing personnel knowledgeable about the job or position who have experience relevant to the subject area. Conduct this data collection method through face-to-face interviews and/or through a survey.
- In the group interview, job performers are assembled to give information relative to their job. The instructional analyst asks questions about job performance and may ask the group to list data on tasks that cannot easily be demonstrated or observed. Because the group interview involves recall rather than recognition, it may provide inaccurate or incomplete data point for task identification.
- The observation/interview method involves sending the instructional analyst to observe and interview job incumbents and their supervisors on the job. Observing the person(s) at work allows flexibility in gathering the required data by providing the instructional analyst opportunities to continually evaluate the information obtained.
- Direct observation of personnel as they perform their job, combined with interviews, provides the most useful source of task information. The instructional analyst should have a thorough understanding of the literature and functional relationships of the job to correctly interpret and describe the behaviors observed.

- In the Subject Matter Experts method, experienced and knowledgeable personnel from various activities are brought together to record and analyze the data on jobs for which many critical behaviors are not directly observable. This method can effectively supplement on-site observation/job analysis and written surveys. The experts are selected for their experience and knowledge of the job.

3) Answer C:

Employee annual performance evaluations should always be based on sound measurable objective criteria which is fully understood by both the supervisor and employee. The rating will be most valuable if the rating is discussed with the employee and directions for improvement are indicated.

4) Answer B:

Brainstorming is a technique of group interactions, often defined as 5-7 members, that encourages each participant to present ideas on a specific issue. The method is normally used to find new, innovative approaches to issues. There are four ground rules:

- Ideas presented are not criticized.
- Freewheeling creative thinking and building on ideas are positively reinforced.
- As many ideas as possible should be presented quickly.
- Combining several ideas or improving suggestions is encouraged.

Brainstorming			
Advantages	Limitations	Uses	Types of Objectives
Interactive Relevant Creative Can be entertaining.	Time consuming. Requires skilled facilitator	Problem solving Trouble shoot Enhanced by pictures/media.	Best for knowledge-level objectives, Problem Solving

5) Answer A:

Some words that should be **avoided** when writing learning objectives are *known*, *understand*, *appreciate*, *learn*, *cover*, *and study*. It is almost impossible to determine if a student has accomplished those objectives. Some example preferred words are **explain**, **classify compare**, **calculate**, **demonstrate**, **operate**, **measure**, **troubleshoot**, **analyze**, **develop**, **and plan**. An example is "each individual will describe in their own works the three primary ISO

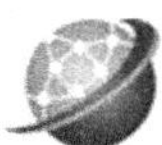

standards that apply to safety management".

6) Answer D:

Training objectives should, above all, be reasonable, measurable and obtainable. It is very desirable, but not imperative that the objectives and goals for any program be written, so as not to be misplaced or relegated to a low priority. When writing training objectives, use action verbs such as add, answer, compare, line up, etc. Avoid words such as understand, know, comprehend and notice as these are actions are difficult to measure. To gain a competitive edge, training must involve more than basic job skills. Included now are advanced skills and understanding of customers and entire manufacturing system. The training is linked to strategic business goals and specific objectives and uses an instructional designed process to ensure effective training which compares favorably with training programs found in other companies.

7) Answer C:

This is the definition of a needs analysis and will help safety inspectors decide between training and non-training needs. The primary question that has to be answered, "Is this a problem that training will resolve or is there a better solution?" After defining the performance discrepancy, instead of training, a new set of work instructions may solve the problem.
An example could be to hang out a PPE required sign to remind personnel that PPE is required when they operate a particular machine. An analytical approach to support the needs analysis would be to complete an operational hazard analysis.

8) Answer C:

Most training experts rate job task analysis as the primary aid in developing course training goals and content.

9) Answer D:

According to Authors Mager, Peterson, Knowles, and many others, a facilitators actions have a major impact on how a learner reacts to the training environment. Usually adults tend not to model behavior that is punished. To avoid conflicting values, safety training objectives should be relevant to the work environment.

10) Answer C:
Learning objectives are always completed before you develop a lesson plan in the design phase.

11) Answer A:
Training should be developed and evaluated based largely on management expectations, employee expectations, and deliver skills and knowledge.
The training program shall be planned and implemented to ensure that:

- Personnel are assigned and supported to ensure adequate program administration and management.
- Budgets are available to fund all elements of the training program.
- Sufficient personnel and expertise are available for the development, delivery, and evaluation of training.

"Competent" means possessing the skills, knowledge, experience, and judgment to perform assigned tasks or activities satisfactorily as determined by the employer. OSHA "competent person" is defined as "one who is capable of identifying existing and predictable hazards in the surroundings or working conditions which are unsanitary, hazardous, or dangerous to employees, and who has authorization to take prompt corrective measures to eliminate them (OSHA). The major motivational condition that best represents the characteristics and skills of a trainer providing effective feedback is Competence. Competency is generally defined in many resources as having the skills, knowledge and abilities to perform a task. A trainer must be competent in facilitation skills and subject matter to be able to provide effective learner feedback. ANSI/ASSE 490.1 defines a Competent Training Professional as a person prepared by education, training, or experience to develop and implement various elements of a training program. Also, known in the standard as a Training Professional.

12) Answer C:
The case study is an especially effective technique for safety and health training since it often illustrates the multi-causal aspects of accidents, as well as the tragic consequences. The case study is an excellent problem-solving technique that *facilitates interactive learning*. Normally case studies are presented to a group that has the goal of evaluating mistakes made in a situation and providing real world solutions. The technique is particularly effective when the group can conclude that they can benefit from mistakes of other organizations and thus prevent accidents.

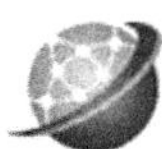

The case study is an excellent tool for developing analytical skills. A major disadvantage to the case study is that a preexisting case may not actually relate to a specific training situation. Common instructional strategies are listed in the table below:

Case Study			
Advantages	Limitations	Uses	Types of Objectives
Interactive Relevant Explore complex issues Applies new knowledge Can be entertaining.	Time consuming. May not see relevance	Develop analytic and problem-solving skills Enhanced by pictures/media.	Best for knowledge-level objectives, Problem Solving

13) Answer C:
The facilitator of adult learning is a guide to adults who are involved in an educational journey. Being technically proficient is not enough, a trainer must possess personality characteristics, interpersonal skills, and positive behaviors. A trainer's attitude is a major motivational condition that has a great impact on creating a conducive learning environment.
Dr. Knowles' theory of andragogy is an attempt to develop a theory specifically for adult learning. Knowles emphasizes that adults are self-directed and expect to take responsibility for decisions. Adult learning programs must accommodate this fundamental aspect.

Andragogy makes the following assumptions about the design of learning:

(1) Adults need to know why they need to learn something
(2) Adults need to learn experientially,
(3) Adults approach learning as problem-solving, and
(4) Adults learn best when the topic is of immediate value.

In practical terms, andragogy means that instruction for adults needs to focus more on the process and less on the content being taught. Strategies such as case studies, role playing, simulations, and self-evaluation are most useful. Instructors adopt a role of facilitator or resource rather than lecturer or grader.

Six Characteristics of Adult Learning:

1) Are Autonomous and self-directed
2) Have a foundation of life experiences and knowledge
3) Are Goal Oriented
4) Are relevancy oriented
5) Are Practical in Nature
6) Need to be shown respect

Four Adult Learning Needs:

1) Need to know why-application to immediate challenges
2) Need to apply experience – opportunity to share and discuss
3) Need to be in control of their learning – Flexible environment, voice concerns
4) Want to learn things that will make them more effective and successful

Adults have four basic training needs:

- Adults need to know why they are learning a particular topic or skill, because the need to apply learning to immediate, real-life challenges.
- Adults have experience that they apply to all new learning.
- Adults need to be in control of their own learning.
- Adults want to learn things that will make them more effective and successful.

To help accomplish these needs, include precise behavioral guidelines and procedures that the trainees are required to follow.

14) Answer C:

Both Quality and OHS management systems are built on the well-known ***Plan-Do-Check-Act*** process. Briefly stated, the purpose of the standards is to provide organizations with an effective tool for continuous improvement in their occupational health and safety management systems to reduce the risk of occupational injuries, illnesses and fatalities. Check is the phase when management verifies that efforts are implemented adequately.

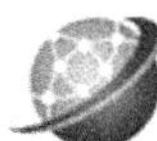

15) Answer A:

Role playing is ideally suited for human relations education or training. It allows students to become participants in a "drama" or "play" that depicts the interaction of humans during stressful or error provocative situations. The technique is **not** suited for problem solving or technical training.

Role Play Strategy			
Advantages	Limitations	Uses	Types of Objectives
Creates a learner-centered environment. Employs learner creativity. Elicits empathy. Addresses complex issues. Can be entertaining.	Participants may be resistant. Risk of embarrassing participants. Easily distracted, difficult to maintain control. Requires intense focused on the objective. Requires a skilled facilitator	Useful as a cap-stone exercise to bring together learned concepts Promotes an understand others' perspective Excellent for active participants.	Excellent for affective and problem-solving exercises.

16) Answer C:

One of the most valuable group techniques is the conference guided discussion. The strength of the guided discussion is in the individual knowledge and experience of the participants. The number of members should be kept small to allow for maximum exchange of ideas. The establishment of goals and objectives is crucial to the success of this method. But more than anything else, this teaching method hinges on the capability of the facilitator or instructor. The facilitator logs the objectives and keeps information and opinions flowing during sessions.

After the discussion, the facilitator distributes recommendations and informs members of actions taken as a result. Shortfalls associated with this method include the trusting a facilitator to ensure that the conference does not become a bull session and recognizing that if management does not follow up on recommendations, then the group will not likely support future efforts.

Guided Discussion Strategy			
Advantages	Limitations	Uses	Types of Objectives
Encourages participation. Shows respect for participants' knowledge. Stimulates interest. Allows instructor to check for understanding. Useful in many situations.	Can be dominated by one individual or faction. Susceptible to drift or "mission creep". Can be difficult to focus on objectives. Can degenerate into a lecture or chaos. Does not give trainer complete control.	Can be used as an icebreaker. Can be used to generate ideas. Can be used to solve problems. Can be used for review. Best to use with small groups – or a large group divided into small groups. Useful for both active participants and reflective observers	Best for comprehension and problem-solving objectives.

17) Answer C:

The valuable attributes of interactive computer-based training (CBT), self-directed learning, distance learning or hybrid or blended learning are as follows:

- Workers can work at their own pace.
- Records of all training can be automatically kept.
- Correct answers are required before a student can proceed.
- Workers receive training as time is available.
- Instructors guide workers step by step through the lesson plan.
- This method works extremely well for organizations with a small workforce or that cannot remove large groups from their jobs at any one time.

Distance learning is an umbrella term for many types of remote learning. Before implementing any type of training, a needs analysis should be completed to ensure that the best method is being selected.

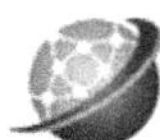

18) Answer B:

Using a variety of strategies or choosing the most appropriate strategy helps trainers accomplish the learning objectives, reach different types of learning styles, and maintain relevance for the learners. The trainer should be able to review the objectives on the training plan and select instructional strategies appropriate for the objectives, the audience, and the conditions.

The scale in increasing order of learning retention includes: Less effective = 1; More effective = 10

1. Words, spoken or written
2. Auditory aids
3. Still pictures
4. Motion pictures
5. Live television
6. Displays
7. Familiarization
8. Demonstration
9. Simulations
10. Actual experience

According to ANSI Z490.1 – 2012 section 4 Training Development, training that will improve the occupational safety, health, or environmental knowledge, skills, or abilities used by the trainees in the performance of their jobs shall be developed. Training development shall follow a systematic process including needs assessment, learning objectives, adult learning principles, course design, and evaluation strategy criteria for completion, and continuous improvement. An important element of an overall training program management system is record keeping and documentation.

Gagné (1985) created a nine-step process called the events of instruction, which correlate to and address the conditions of learning:

1. Gaining attention: To ensure reception of coming instruction, the teacher gives the learners a stimulus. Before the learners can start to process any new information, the instructor must gain the attention of the learners. This might entail using abrupt changes in the instruction.
2. Informing learners of objectives: The teacher tells the learner what they will be able to do because of the instruction. The teacher communicates the desired outcome to the group.
3. Stimulating recall of prior learning: The teacher asks for recall of existing relevant knowledge.
4. Presenting the stimulus: The teacher gives emphasis to distinctive features.
5. Providing learning guidance: The teacher helps the students in understanding (semantic encoding) by providing organization and relevance.

6. Eliciting performance: The teacher asks the learners to respond, demonstrating learning.
7. Providing feedback: The teacher gives informative feedback on the learners' performance.
8. Assessing performance: The teacher requires more learner performance, and gives feedback, to reinforce learning.
9. Enhancing retention and transfer: The teacher provides varied practice to generalize the capability.

19) Answer B:

The target audience is the group of learners. A good training needs analysis provides the trainer with intelligence about target audience demographics. Relevant details such as:

- Educational background
- Level of experience with the training topic
- Job Duties and responsibilities
- Risk factors
- History of training
- Length of employment
- Organizational climate
- Attitudes toward training
- Mastery of prerequisite skills/knowledge/abilities
- Medical requirements

Through audience analysis, the trainer can adjust in the instructional strategies to meet learner needs and performance objectives. Adjustments can vary from peer groups or individuals; the purpose is that they can accomplish the learning objective. Selecting the media for delivering instructional content should be done only after a planning process.

1) Determining if Training is Needed
2) Identifying Training Needs
3) Identifying Goals and Objectives
4) Developing Learning Activities
5) Conducting the Training
6) Evaluating Program Effectiveness
7) Improving the Program

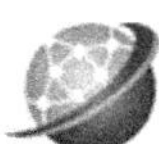

Systems Approach to Training and Instructional Systems Design Models

Analysis
Needs Assessment
Select Analysis method
Plan Analysis
Identify Target Audience
Perform Analysis
Select job/task content for instruction
Construct Performance Measures
Analyze existing materials
Select instruction and environment
Design
Develop Objectives
Develop Tests or test items
Develop Prerequisites
Determine Sequence and structure
Development
Specify learning events/activities
Specify Delivery Methods
Develop Management plan
Review/select/modify existing materials
Develop instructional materials/methods & other interventions
Validate/pilot instruction or intervention
Implementation
Implement instructional management plan
Provide exceptions and test-out options
Conduct instruction or implement intervention
Evaluation
Internal Program Reactions, Behavior, and Performance
External Supervision Job Performance indicators
Validation Control of Quality Revision

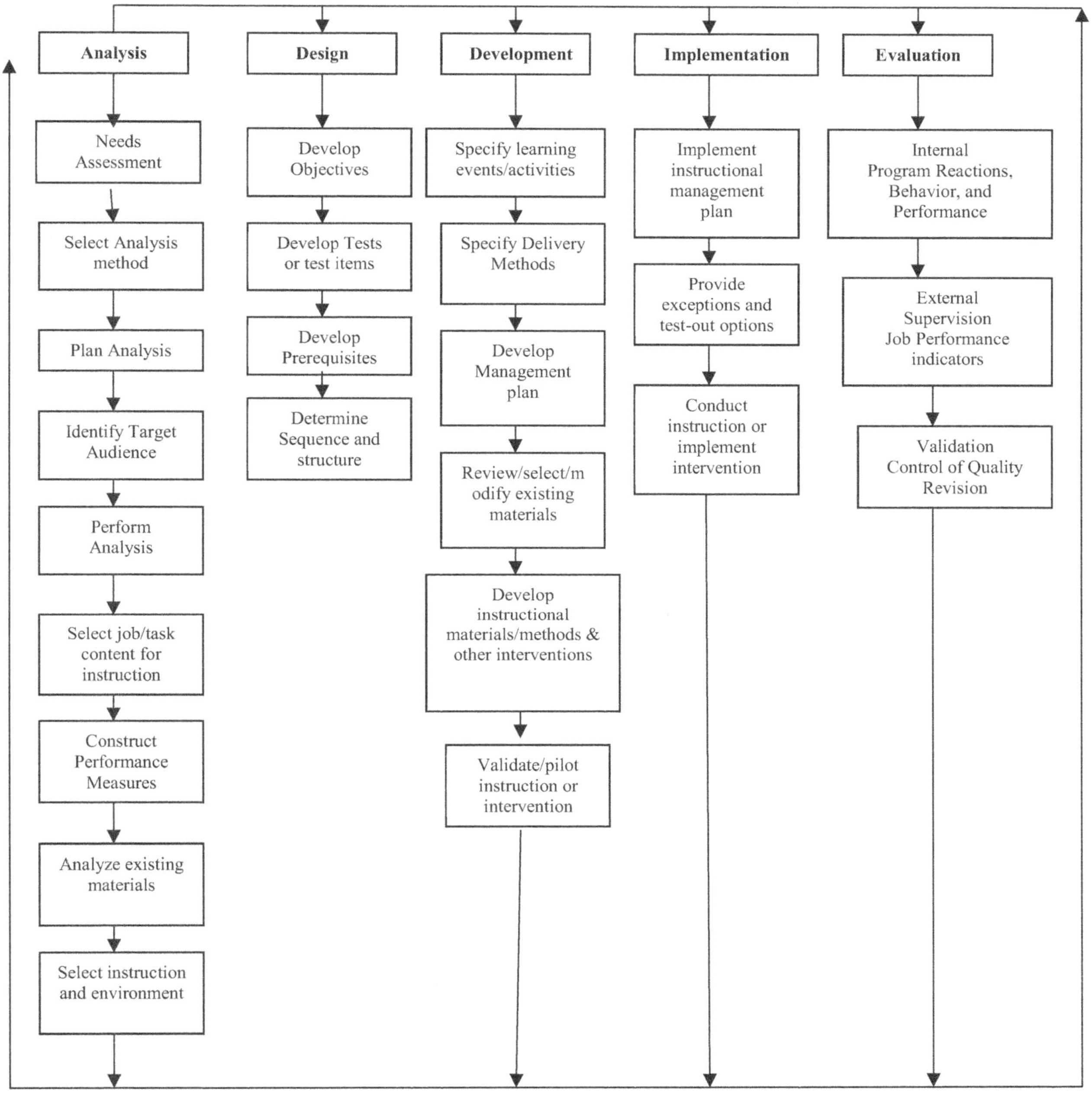

20) Answer A:

During any training situation when attempting to change habits or procedures, the trainee will have questions as to why it is necessary and why the recommended way best. When the trainee is permitted to share ideas, evaluate the material and become involved, their overall acceptance of course material will increase.

Domain 1 Quiz 3 Questions

1) Successful adult learning is evaluated **least effectively** by:
   A) Learner demonstrating application of knowledge.
   B) Instructor providing a video of a previous experience.
   C) Observing the learner practice a new skill.
   D) Discussing feedback with the supervisor about how new skills have improved performance.

2) A supervisor is conducting training on the use of air-purifying respirators to several crews of disaster site workers. For progrm reliability, it is ***most*** important for the trainer to:
   A) Dress for the occasion.
   B) Become a subject matter expert on respirators.
   C) Use an abundance of visual aids.
   D) Use a well-prepared lesson plan.

3) The **primary** benefit of safety training is:
   A) Reduction of production costs.
   B) Improved employee performance.
   C) Fewer incidents/accidents.
   D) Reinforcement of operational organization goals.

4) During a training needs assessment does **not** include:
   A) Development of instructional strategies.
   B) Identity the problem or need before designing a solution.
   C) Cost benefit analysis of training solutions.
   D) Evaluate the impact of a training solution before development.

5) The main elements in the ANSI Z490.1 training standard for effective safety and health training program include
   A) Evaluation, development, delivery, program management, documentation.
   B) Scope, needs assessment, management commitment, recordkeeping.
   C) Employee involvement, training checklist, management accountability, trainer qualifications.
   D) Delivery, learning objectives, management evaluation, annexes

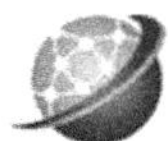

6) On the third day of a five-day course, a new trainer arrives to teach the remainder of the class. The trainer identifies that two of the people seated next to each are being disruptive. The **first** option for managing the disruptive behavior is:

  A) Identify the disruptive persons to the entire class before the next break, warn if the behavior continues they will be removed and senior management will be notified by email.
  B) Arbitrarily rearrange the entire class seating placements during break to separate the disruptive students.
  C) Make eye contact, move towards the disruptive behavior, and if the behavior continues, speak privately with the disruptive persons at a break, seeking resolution.
  D) Make an example of the disruptive person by making them stand in the back of the room, explaining to the class that disruption won't be tolerated.

7) Which situation would **likely** require a solution other than safety training?

  A) Worker refuses to follow safety rules.
  B) Workers that are new hires.
  C) Experienced worker transferring to a new job.
  D) New procedures will be implemented.

8) An effective safety training program must have the following components; performance based, established implementation plan, measured, and:

  A) Apply to both individual and group settings.
  B) Use audio-visual presentations supported by printed materials.
  C) Transfer knowledge prior to hazardous exposures.
  D) Delivered only by specially trained and highly skilled instructors.

9) The **first** phase in designing a successful a safety training program is to:

  A) Design learning objectives.
  B) Conduct a training needs assessment.
  C) Develop instructional strategies.
  D) Plan for a conducive learning environment.

10) The management of change process involves the identification of hazards associated with the change; assessment of the risks associated with the change; consideration of the hazards and risks prior to the change; and
   A) Implementation of controls needed to address hazards and risks associated with the change.
   B) Performance of a "what if" analysis to identify expected risks of the proposed change.
   C) Expand safety staff to oversee and management of the change.
   D) Document compliance with all applicable regulatory guide lines regarding changes in the OHSMS.

11) The training implementation phase includes instructor costs, student costs, materials costs, and:
   A) Facilities costs.
   B) Curriculum development costs.
   C) Recordkeeping costs.
   D) Marketing costs.

12) The training method that provides the **most** information retention is:
   A) Reading.
   B) Listening.
   C) Active.
   D) Seeing.

13) Which training is **most** appropriate for supervisors?
   A) Training in the safe use of products.
   B) Training in doing a job correctly and safely.
   C) Training when the job changes.
   D) Training in hazards and controls.

14) According to ANSI Z10 management systems should demonstrate leadership as a core organizational value and establish effective employee participation by seeking to:
   A) Provide obstacles that enhance communication barriers.
   B) Minimizing labor representation.
   C) Dictating safety as a the condition of employment.
   D) Identify and remove communication barriers.

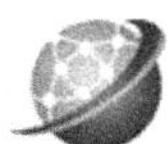

15) Training and education are often used interchangeably but have different meanings. The **major** distinction between training and education is:
   A) Education focuses on learning about and training focuses on learning how.
   B) Training focuses on learning about and education focuses on learning how.
   C) Education is more focused on application of skills and training is focused on building knowledge.
   D) Training develops knowledge for future use and education provides relevant skills for immediate use.

16) You are facilitating a one hour training session and arrive five minutes before the start of class to find that your presentation did not synchronize with the company server. Participants are taking their seats and you do not have access to the presentation. What is the **best** course of action?
   A) Cancel the training session.
   B) Reschedule the training session for a later time.
   C) Get into your facilitator toolkit and begin the training.
   D) Ask a participant familiar with the topic to deliver the training.

17) Story telling is a useful training strategy to bring context to a situation. The **most** important aspect of the story that it must be:
   A) Factual.
   B) Relevant.
   C) From personal experience.
   D) Humorous.

18) Training is needed for a new process rollout. The training program has been designed, materials are appropriate and purchased, and the training has been conducted. What is remains to be completed?
   A) Learning objectives.
   B) Program evaluation.
   C) Curriculum design.
   D) Needs analysis.

19) Which training methods allows for the **least** amount of student-instructor interaction?
   A) Lecture.
   B) Role playing.
   C) Case study.
   D) Facilitated discussion.

20) What is **most** important when facilitating individualized instruction as part of a self-directed, distance learning strategy?
   A) Ensure technical competency of the learner.
   B) Control the progress to meet the learning objectives.
   C) Evaluate knowledge gained through standardized testing.
   D) Know the learner's knowledge gaps.

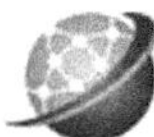

Domain 1 Quiz 3 Answers

1) Answer B:

Adults want satisfactory answers to the following questions to accept and apply learning.

1.) Why is it important?
2.) How can I apply it?
3.) How does it work?
4.) What do I need to know?

The concept of a learning curve is best described as "the level of proficiency tends to reach a limit as the time devoted to learning a task increases".

2) Answer D:

The use of a lesson plan will provide standardization to a presentation and avoid omission of essential material. The lesson plan also helps the instructor conduct the class according to a timetable and should provide for student participation or involvement. Presenting technical information requires training and practice. The effectiveness of a technical presentation depends upon the trainee as well as the instructor. The trainees will be much more open to learning if the instructor succeeds in eliciting a sense of disequilibrium among the trainees.

3) Answer B

According to the NSC, the goal of effective training is learning that leads to improved on-the-job performance. Other benefits include reduction in rejected production items, improvement in housekeeping and lowering the number of preventable accidents. After a training program has been conducted, what is actually applied on the job will be influenced most by the expectations of superiors, peers and subordinates.

4) Answer A:

According to the NSC, a needs assessment helps to

- Distinguish between training and non-training needs
- Identify the problem or need before designing a solution
- Save time and money by ensuring that solutions effectively address problems they are intended to solve
- Identify factors that will impact training before its development

After the needs assessment, training goals are developed and during that process candidates will determine what knowledge the trainee needs to know to eliminate the problem.

5) Answer A:

The ANSI/ASSE Z490.1 on Criteria for Accepted Practices in Safety, Health and Environmental Training includes elements of **training development, delivery, evaluation, and management of training and training programs.** The criteria were developed by combining accepted practices in the training industry with those in the safety, health, and environmental industries and it is intended to apply universally to training programs.

Overview of the ASSE/ANSI Z490.1-2016

1) Scope, Purpose and Application
2) Definitions
3) Management of a Comprehensive Training Program
    a) Accountability & Responsibility
    b) Minimum Training Requirements
    c) Resource Management and Administration
    d) Program Evaluation
4) Training Program/Course Development
    a) Training Development
    b) Needs Assessment
    c) Learning Objectives
    d) Course Design
    e) Evaluation Strategy
    f) Criteria for Completion
    g) Continuous Improvement of the Training Course
5) Training Delivery
    a) Trainer Qualifications
    b) Training Delivery Methods and Materials
6) Training Evaluation
    a) General Criteria
    b) Evaluation Approaches
    c) Continuous Improvement
7) Documentation and Recordkeeping
    a) Systems and Procedure
    b) Records
    c) Record Confidentiality and Availability
    d) Issuing Certificates
8) Annexes:
    a) Annex A References
    b) Annex B Training Course Development Guidelines
    c) Annex C Safety, Health and Environmental Trainer's Checklist
    d) Annex D Virtual Learning

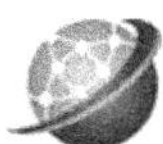

6) Answer C:

Setting classroom expectations at the very beginning of a class is one of the best methods of classroom management. Hang a flip chart or poster, or dedicate a section of white board if you have the space, and list expected classroom behaviors. Refer to this list when disruptions occur. Using a flip chart or white board can be especially useful because you can involve students in the construction of the list on the first day and in that way get buy-in. Start with a few of your own expectations and ask the group for additional suggestions. When all agree on how the classroom is to be managed, disruptions are minimal.

A list of expectations may include:

- Set the tone: "We are all Adults and Professionals…"
- Start and end on time
- Turn off or silence cell phones
- Save texting for breaks
- Respect the contributions of others
- Be open to new ideas
- Resolve differences calmly
- Stay on topic

Unless you've got a purposefully disruptive student in your classroom, disruptions, are likely to be minimal. We're talking about disruptions like chatting in the back of the room, texting, or someone who is argumentative or disrespectful. Try one, or more, if necessary, of the following tactics:

- Make eye contact with the disruptive person
- Remind the group of the agreed-upon norms
- Move toward the disruptive person
- Stand directly in front of the person
- Be silent and wait for the disruption to end
- Acknowledge the input, put it in your "parking lot" if appropriate, and keep moving forward to meet the learning objectives.
    - "You may be right."
    - "Thanks for your comment."
    - "How about if we park that comment and come back to it later."
- Ask for help from the group
    - "What does everyone else think?"
- Call for a break and speak with the person(s) privately seeking resolution.
- Rearrange the seating as part of a learning activity.

For more serious problems, or if the disruption persists:

- Call for a break and speak with the person(s) privately seeking resolution.
- Confront the behavior, not the person
- Speak for yourself only, not the class
- Seek to understand the reason for the disruption
- Ask the person to recommend a solution
- Review your expectations of classroom behavior if necessary
- Try to get agreement on expected norms
- Explain any consequences of continued disruptions

7) Answer A:

Safety training the right solution to a performance problem involving the lack of skills, knowledge or abilities. However, training is not intended to correct performance issues such as a worker refusing to follow safety rules.

8) Answer C:

To design an effective training program, the safety professional must focus on the learners needs, analyze learner characteristics, develop specific learning objectives, create materials and schedules, and design appropriate testing and evaluation methods. The main goal is to transfer knowledge about workplace hazards before a worker is exposed to those hazards.

9) Answer B:

To create an effective training program, first the safety professional needs to assess current worker performance, comparing it to the desired performance. Planning and development of training begin with an understanding of how people learn and what contributes to learning. The following list summarizes some principles of learning.

- *Stimulate multiple senses*. We receive most information through vision. Hearing processes a lot of information, but cannot handle information at the same rate as visual input. Incorporating visual materials into training helps the learning process.
- *Identify the need for training*. The trainee will understand what is being learned better if objectives and strategy for training are presented clearly.

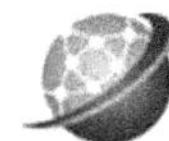

- *Organize the content logically.* It is better to conduct training in small modules rather than large ones. What constitutes logical order depends on the material being taught. One form of order is proper sequence, where early modules establish the background for later modules. Another form of order is level of difficulty, where easy material progresses to that which is more difficult.
- *Teach principles with procedures.* People will understand procedures better and retain them longer if the principle or objective for the procedures is presented first.
- *Teach the whole process first, then detailed parts.* Trainees should learn the whole procedure first. They need to see what each step leads to. Then they can go through the details of the process.
- *Make sure trainees have time to practice, but keep practice periods short.* When trainees are learning skills and the criterion for success is meeting some performance standard, trainees need time to practice. Short practice periods with breaks are more effective than long practice sessions.
- *Ensure participation when performance is the goal.* When training occurs in group arrangements, some trainees hold back from participating. An instructor must watch for this and find ways to involve everyone
- *Give trainees knowledge of results.* Trainees need to know how they are doing. It is better to evaluate trainees in small increments and give them results of evaluations, rather than delay evaluation and results.
- *Reward correct performance.* There are many forms of feedback. Positive is generally better than negative. Praise and verbal comments can be used when trainees do things correctly. Accurate and immediate feedback is better than delayed and general feedback.
- *Keep trainees interested and challenged.* Instructors can use various techniques to increase participation and interest in subject materials. Ask questions and stimulate discussion, and when there are skills involving several people, role playing exercises help maintain interest.
- *Simulation should duplicate actual conditions.* When procedures and settings are simulated, they should accurately represent real situations as much as possible. Unrealistic simulation can lead to incorrect behavior in real contexts.

- *Unique or unusual material is retained longest*. Use of examples and real situations helps people visualize what is taught. Dramatic and exotic style may be entertaining, but care must be given to make sure such activity is meaningful.
- *Provide relearning to sustain knowledge and skill*. The idea of a learning curve tells us that the more skilled a person becomes, the slower the rate of improvement. After training, the knowledge or skill achieved by the end of training decays with time. Creating opportunities to relearn, update, or evaluate skills and knowledge will help keep performance at desired levels.
- *Fit training to individual needs*. The knowledge or skill of each trainee can be assessed through pretests, interviews, and other evaluations. When there is too great a range in knowledge and skill in the same training session, few trainees are well served. With self-paced instruction and criterion-based training, individuals can achieve the desired level of knowledge or skill at their own pace. Slow learners or those with elementary skills are not intimidated by others who are advanced. Computer based instruction and training systems allow for customized instruction and repeating of sessions to match the needs of individuals.

10) Answer A:
The management of change process covers four primary concepts, regardless of the type of change (Kausek, 2007):

- Identification of hazard s associated with the change
- Assessment of the risks associated with the change
- Consideration of the hazards and risks prior to the change
- Implementation of controls needed to address hazards and risks associated with the change

Management of change is the process to identify and managme changes to minimize the introduction of new hazatrds and risks into the work environmental. Examples include changes in technology, equipment, facilities, work practices and procedures, design specifications, raw materials, organizational staffing changes, and standards or regulations(ANSI Z10-2012).

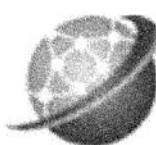

Management of change shall include:

- Identification of tasks and related health and safety hazards
- Recognition of hazards associated with human factors including human errors caused by design deficiencies
- Review of applicable regulations, codes, standards, internal and external recognized guidelines.
- Application of control measures (Hierarchy of controls)
- A dtermination of the appropriate scope and degree of the design revewi and management of change
- Employee participation

Integrating the change analysis concept within the management of change process is to assure that:

- Hazards and risks that may arise are identified and assessed (risk assessment) and that appropriate control measures are taken.
- New hazards created are controlled to an acceptable risk.
- Previously resolved hazards are not negatively impacted-increasing the risk.
- The OHSMS is not negatively impacted.

11) Answer A:

Safety training costs can be broken down into three major categories - development, implementation, and other lifecycle costs. Development costs include curriculum development and materials. Implementation costs include instructor cost, student cost, material cost and facility cost. Other life cycle costs include recordkeeping and training evaluations, revisions, software licensing and maintenance fees, information technology support, internal salaries.

12) Answer C:

Active training can be defined as a two-way interactive learning processes with continual feedback, to achieve the purpose of the learning objective(s) Active Training is a method of education that uses unconventional means to motivate students to become more involved, physically & mentally, in applying material/content. Active training is an effective teaching method that takes into account different learning styles and social components. Characteristics include:

- Learning by doing/ hands-on
- Contingent (step-by-step)
- Individual has control over what/ how much they learn
- Facilitates participation

Demonstration/ Practice Strategy			
Advantages	Limitations	Uses	Types of Objectives
Provides hands-on experience/practice. Incorporates multiple senses and learning styles Proficiency evaluated through demonstrated performance	Requires significant preparation. Is time consuming. May increase safety risks. May require a cadre of instructors.	Useful for any hands-on skills. Useful for trouble-shooting. Works well only with small groups. Excellent for active participants.	Best with application-level/psychomotor objectives Useful for problem-solving with equipment (trouble-shooting)

13) Answer D:
Supervisors and managers represent company and employer responsibilities. Not only do they need to understand the hazards and controls for their workers, but they need to know what training they must administer. They need to understand the regulatory and legal responsibilities for safety that the employer or company bears and they need to know what responsibilities they have under normal and special procedures. If supervisors and managers have contract relationships with other companies and their employees, the supervisors and managers must learn how to deal with safety matters through contract chains of command.

14) Answer D:
The ANSI Z10 Occupational Health and Safety Management Systems (OHSMS) standard provides guidelines for how organizations should establish a process to ensure effective employee participation at all levels. Leadership begins with top management providing the directive for integrating health and safety into the daily functions of the business. Leadership by top management communicates safety as a core value and engenders trust through "walking the talk". Leadership should identify and remove obstacles or barriers to participation in the OHSMS. Employees performing work tasks can contribute valuable insight. Management should encourage employee participation in the design, implementation, and ongoing operations of the OHSMS. Participation in:

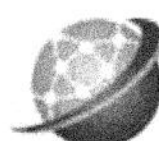

- Hazard reviews and job safety analysis
- Incident investigations
- Health and safety committees
- Development of training programs
- Risk assessments, inspections and audits
- Selection of PPE
- Recognition and involvement programs

15) Answer A:
Training is more immediate, skills oriented, and focused on application as compared to education, which is the process of building a base of knowledge. In OHS both strategies are important. Organizations often focus on skills based or traditional training. Training in hazard communication typically might focus on how to read an SDS and labels, handle workplace chemicals, etc. Education in hazard communication could focus on historical perspective, and on examining case studies of OSHA fines or major chemical exposure events.

16) Answer C:
First, facilitators should arrive early, at least 30 minutes before the start of training to get set up (mentally and technologically), check the learning environment, verify materials are in order, and greet participants as they arrive. It is always a good idea to carry a backup memory stick with a copy of the presentation. To be an effective trainer/facilitator, one must have a go-to facilitator toolkit. While multi-media presentations are great tools, death by power point is the result of this technology being overused as a crutch for poor facilitation skills. Some of the best presentations delivered by skilled facilitators have been out of spontaneity due to technical difficulties. On the other hand, such disruption can be disastrous for a one dimensional, inflexible, or novice instructor. Bottom line: Have a backup plan. One of the pitfalls of instruction is that trainers tend to develop training programs that accommodate the way the trainer learns best, not the way the participants learn best. The key to accommodating learning styles is that instructional strategies and media should be selected as a means to help the learner and not as a convenience for the instructor. The best training stimulates multiple senses in the learner and should be a blend various learning strategies:

  - Lecture
  - Brain Storm
  - Case Study
  - Demonstration

- Role Play
- Guided Discussion
- Self-Directed/Distance Learning
- Learner Discovery/Individualized instruction
- Interactive Computer-Based Training (CBT)
- Activity based-Hands On/Demonstration
- e-learning/m-learning
- Hybrid/blended

Many people recognize that each person prefers different learning styles and techniques. Learning styles group common ways that people learn. Everyone has a mix of learning styles. Some people may find that they have a dominant style of learning, with far less use of the other styles. Others may find that they use different styles in different circumstances. There is no right mix. Nor are your styles fixed. You can develop ability in less dominant styles, as well as further develop styles that you already use well. Giving consideration to learning styles helps trainers to:

- Recognize that everyone learns differently and the need for a variety of instructional strategies and media.
- Recognize that trainers ***also*** have preferred learning styles.
- Learner focus, not instructor focus.
- Be creative and include exercises or instructional strategies or media that help adults learn the information and appropriate for the learning objectives.
- Make real time adjustments and employ alternative instructional methods best suited to the learners and accomplish the learning objectives.
- Empathize with training participants.

By recognizing and understanding learning styles, skilled trainers can use a variety of techniques best suited to the audience and learning objectives. This improves the speed and quality of training.

The ANSI Z490-2009 Criteria for Accepted Practices in Safety, Health and Environmental Training is a well-constructed standard specific to SH&E training.

Competency is having the skills, knowledge and abilities to perform the task as determined by the employer.

Competent Training Professional is a person prepared by education, training, or experience to develop and implement various elements of a training

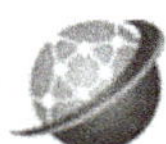

program. Also known in the Z490 standard as a Training Professional.
Trainer is the person who delivers a training event.
Trainer Criteria represents the criteria for safety, health, and environmental trainers shall be specified during training development. Criteria shall include subject matter expertise and training delivery skills.

17) Answer B:
According to Authors Mager, Peterson, Knowles, and many others, a facilitators actions have a major impact on how a learner reacts to the training environment. Adult learners are relevancy oriented, pragmatic, and interested in the immediate application of knowledge, i.e., the "so what" factor. Author Elain Biech in *Training and Development for Dummies* (2015), explains storytelling as telling an event (true or fictitious) that has a moral or lesson, or demonstrated consequences. The punch line leaves the listener inspired, influenced, or improved, without explaining the learning point. The most important factor of storytelling as a facilitator is to be relevant to the audience and learning objectives.

18) Answer B:
The ADDIE instructional design model is the generic process traditionally used by instructional designers and training developers. The ADDIE model is at the very core of instructional design and is the basis of instructional systems design (ISD). There are various adaptations of the ADDIE model but it generally consists of five cyclical phases:

1. Analysis
2. Design
3. Development
4. Implementation
5. Evaluation.

These processes represent a dynamic, flexible guideline for building effective training and performance support tools. Most current ISD models are variations of the ADDIE process. Rapid prototyping is a commonly accepted improvement to this model. This is the idea of reviewing continual or formative feedback while creating instructional materials. This model strives to save time and money by catching problems while they are still easy to fix.

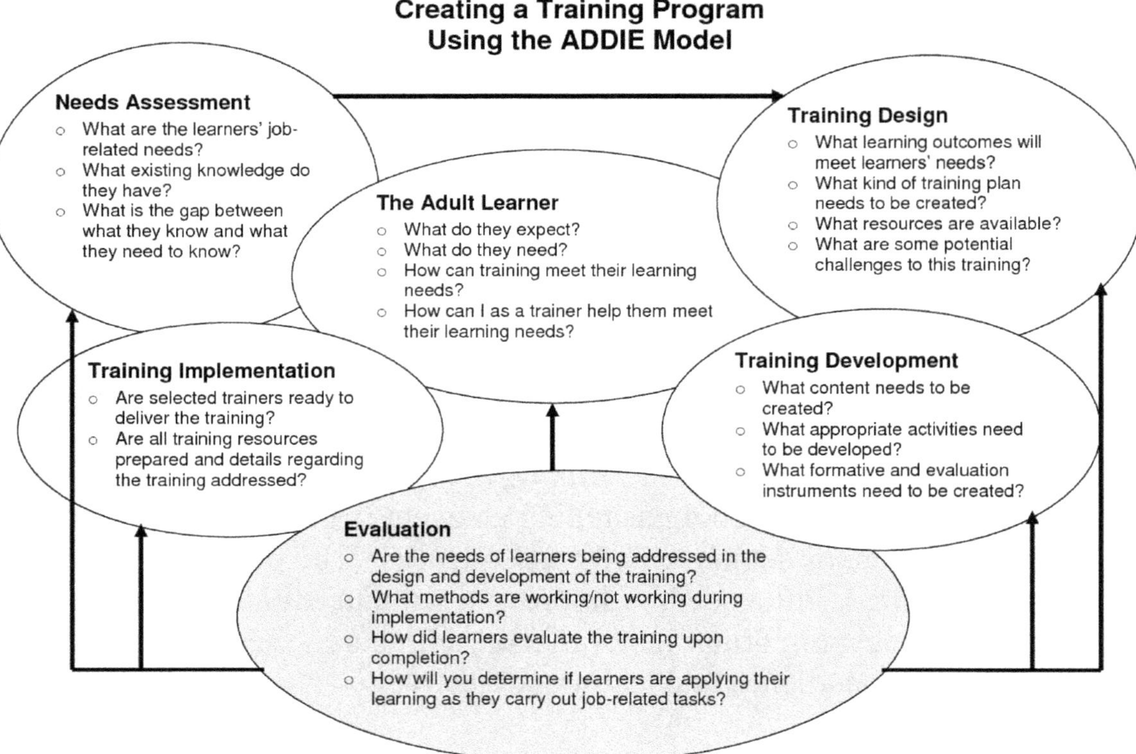

19) Answer A:
The benefit of lecture is that information can be imparted to a large group in a relatively short time. However, this leaves little time or opportunity for interaction between trainee and instructor.

Lecture Strategy			
Advantages	Limitations	Uses	Types of Objectives
Presents much information in a short time. Provides for instructor control. Good for introducing and summarizing new information. Can be entertaining.	Does not develop reasoning skills. Makes learners dependent on instructor. Is instructor-paced. Tends to be over-used. Can be boring.	Introduce new material. To summarize lesson. To establish instructor's expertise and leadership. Excellent for reflective observers. Enhanced by media.	Best for knowledge-level objectives, acquisition of facts.

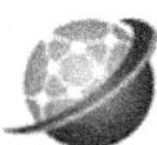

20) Answer D:

Self-directed learning involves having employees take responsibility for all aspects of learning-when it is conducted and who will be involved. Learners master predetermined training content at their own pace without an instructor. Trainers may serve as facilitators. That is, trainers are available to evaluate learning or answer questions for the trainee. The trainer does not control or disseminate instruction. The learning process is controlled by the learner. There are several advantages and disadvantages of self-directed learning. It allows trainees to learn at their own pace and receive feedback about the learning performance. For the company, self-directed learning requires fewer trainers, reduces costs associated with travel and meeting rooms, and makes multiple-site training more realistic. Self-directed learning provides consistent training content that captures the knowledge of experts. Self-directed learning also makes it easier for shift employees to gain access to training materials. Self-directed learning is likely to become more common in the future as companies seek to train staff flexibly, take advantage of technology, and encourage employees to be proactive in their learning rather than driven by the employer. A major disadvantage of self-directed learning is that trainees must be willing and comfortable learning on their own. That is, trainees must be motivated to learn. From the company perspective, self-directed learning results in higher development costs, and development time is longer than with other types of training programs.

Several steps are necessary to develop effective self-directed learning:

1. Conducting a job analysis to identify the tasks that must be covered.
2. Writing trainee-centered learning objectives directly related to the tasks. Because the objectives take the place of the instructor, they must indicate what information is important, what actions the trainee should take, and what the trainee should master.
3. Developing the content for the learning package. This involves developing scripts (for video) or text screens (for computer-based training). The content should be based on the trainee-centered learning objectives. Another consideration in developing the content is the media (e.g., paper, video, computer, World Wide Web site) that will be used to communicate the content.
4. Breaking the content into smaller pieces ("chunks"). The chunks should always begin with the objectives that will be covered and include a method for trainees to evaluate their learning. Practice exercises should also appear in each chunk.
5. Developing an evaluation package. This should include evaluation of the trainee and evaluation of the self-directed learning package. Trainee evaluation should be based on the objectives (a process known as criterion referencing). That is, questions should be developed that are written directly from the objectives and can be answered directly from the materials. Evaluation of the self-directed learning package should involve determining ease of use, how up-to-date the material is, if the package is being used as intended, and whether trainees are mastering the objectives.

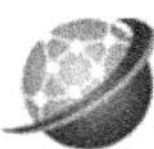

Domain 2: Risk Management

Domain 2: Risk Management 17.1%
Knowledge of: 1. Resources for hazard prevention and control management (e.g., external resources, internal resources, industry standards, subject matter experts) 2. Work planning and controls (e.g., job safety analysis, preliminary hazard analysis, job/task hazard analysis, safe work permit) 3. Prevention through Design concepts (e.g., managing safety through the lifecycle of the program) 4. Common liability exposures (e.g., tort, joint liability, attractive nuisance) 5. Common types of insurance coverage (e.g., differences between property and liability coverage) 6. Hierarchy of controls (e.g., elimination, engineering, substitutions)
Skill to: 1. Interpret and apply information related to hazard prevention and control management (e.g., internal resources, external resources, industry standards, safety data sheet) 2. Identify safety, health, and environmental risk (e.g., checklists, brainstorming, observation, lessons learned, experience, HAZID, process safety) 3. Analyze safety, health, and environmental risk (e.g., severity and likelihood/frequency matrix, historical information, industry data, “what if” analysis, process safety) 4. Evaluate and prioritize safety, health, and environmental risk (e.g., high/low risk) 5. Review and refine implemented safety, health, environmental controls to ensure they are effective 6. Use a risk matrix 7. Apply the hierarchy of controls to various types of hazards while considering the likelihood and severity

Hazard Identification and Risk Assessment

Risk assessment is the process to determine the level of risk based on the likelihood the hazard will cause injury or illness, and the severity of the injury or illness that may result. When a hazard is identified and he potential for harm is discussed, and the probability an incident or exposure can occur, a risk assessment has been conducted. For less complex hazards and risks, the assessment may be based entirely on knowledge and experience. The following definitions are from the ANSI Z10-2012, Occupational Health and Safety Management Systems.

- **Hazard:** A condition, set of circumstances, or inherent property that can cause injury, illness, or death.
  Exposure: Contact with or proximity to a hazard, taking into account duration and intensity.
- **Risk:** An estimate of the combination of the likelihood of an occurrence of a hazardous event or exposure(s), and the severity of injury or illness that may be caused by the event or exposures
- **Probability:** The likelihood of a hazard causing an incident or exposure that could result in harm or damage-for a selected unit of time, events, population, items or activity being considered.
- **Severity:** The extent of harm or damage that could result from a hazard-related incident or exposures.
- **Risk assessment:** Process (es) used to evaluate the level of risk associated with hazards and system issues.

Risk assessment outcomes are used to determine the relative levels of occupational risk and the importance of developing strategies for risk reduction. It is generally acknowledged that zero risk is practically unattainable, and a certain measure of residual risk always remains.

"Safe" can be interpreted as having reached a level of acceptable or minimal residual risk. By identifying acceptable levels of risk, management can best operationalize risk reduction strategies.

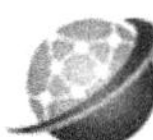

According to ANSI Z10-2012, the following represents a general process of risk assessment:

- Assure Management commitment, involvement and direction
- Select a risk assessment team, including employees with knowledge of jobs and tasks.
- Establish the analysis parameters.
- Select a risk assessment technique.
- Identify the hazards.
- Consider failure modes.
- Assess the severity of consequences.
- Determine occurrence probability, prominently taking into consideration the exposures.
- Define the initial risk.
- Make risk acceptance or non-acceptance decisions with employee involvement.
- If needed, select and implement hazard avoidance, elimination, reduction and control measures.
- Address the residual risk.
- Make risk acceptance or non-acceptance decisions with employee involvement.
- Document the results.
- Follow-up on the actions taken.

The goal of a risk assessment process is to achieve safe working conditions with an acceptable level of risk. There is no single, absolute definition for acceptable risk and it will vary by organization. In general terms, acceptable risk is risk that has been assessed and controlled to a level that is tolerated by the organization. Obtaining zero risk is nearly impossible as there is always residual risk when operations continue.

There are several risk assessment techniques and the method depends on the complexity of the situation.

Risk assessments may include:

- **Accident/incident investigation**: Although reactive it is another tool for uncovering hazards and management system failures. The primary purpose of the accident/incident investigation is to prevent future occurrences. Therefore, the results of the investigation should be used to initiate corrective action.
- **Brain Storming:** A free flowing group discussion by employees who perform a task to identify hazards, risks, and solutions.
- **Job Safety Analysis** (Job Hazard Analysis): A method that can be used to identify, analyze and record the steps involved in performing a specific job; the existing or potential safety and health hazards associated with each step; and the recommended action(s)/procedure(s) that will eliminate or reduce these hazards and the risk of a workplace injury or illness.
- **Trend Analysis:** Worksite Analysis is analysis of injury and illness trends over time, so that patterns with common causes can be identified and prevented. Review of the OSHA injury and illness forms is the most common form of pattern analysis, but other records of hazards can be analyzed for patterns. Examples are inspection records and employee hazard reporting records.
- **What-if:** For relatively uncomplicated processes, review the process from raw materials to product. At each handling or processing step, "what if" questions are formulated and answered, to evaluate the effects of component failures or procedural errors on the process.
- **Checklist**: For more complex processes, the "what if" study can be best organized through the use of a "checklist," and assigning certain aspects of the process to the committee members having the greatest experience or skill in evaluating those aspects. Operator practices and job knowledge are audited in the field, the suitability of equipment and materials of construction is studied, and the chemistry of the process and the control systems are reviewed, and the operating and maintenance records are audited. Generally, a checklist evaluation of a process precedes use of the more sophisticated methods described below, unless the process has been operated safely for many years and has been subjected to periodic and thorough safety inspections and audits.

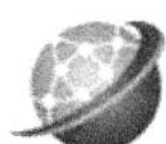

- **What-If/Checklist:** The what-if/checklist is a broadly based hazard assessment technique that combines the creative thinking of a selected team of specialists with the methodical focus of a prepared checklist. The result is a comprehensive hazard analysis that is extremely useful in training operation personnel on the hazards of the particular operation.
- **Failure modes and effects analysis (FMEA):** System analysis technique that identifies the manner in which failures occur and investigates their impact on one another, as well as on other parts of the system.
- **Fault-tree analysis (FTA)**: System safety technique using deductive (general to specific) analysis that starts with an undesired event and analyzes the way the undesired event can occur. Uses Boolean algebra to simplify the fault-tree diagram to a minimal cut set, which is the shortest, most direct path that allows an event to take place.
- **Hazard and operability study (HAZOP)**: Study used to identify problems associated with potential hazards and deviations in plant operations from the design specifications and is carried out by a multidisciplinary team following a structure that includes a series of guide words.
- **Management oversight and risk tree (MORT)**: Analytical system that develops a logic tree to identify total system risks, both those inherent in physical equipment and processes and those arising from operational/management inadequacies.
- **Preliminary hazard analysis (PHA)**: System safety technique that is the initial effort to identify potentially hazardous components within a system during the design phase.
- **Systems hazard analysis (SHA)**: Method that seeks to identify physical and functional incompatibilities between adjacent, interconnected, and interacting elements.
- **System safety engineering report (SSER)**: Report that consists of a compilation of the production phase inputs that identifies and documents the hazards of the final product or system and provides definite conclusions about the safety integrity of the product and the manner in which specific hazards have been controlled.

- **System safety program plan (SSPP)**: Plan that identifies the tasks to be accomplished in the total safety program for the evolution of the system and is considered the key to a successful program.
- **Technique of human rate error prediction (THREP)**: System safety technique that calculates the probability of human operating errors.

Examples of Information Sources for Hazard Identification and Assessment

Source	Description
Equipment and machinery manufacturers	Owner and operator manuals typically include (1) warnings of hazards that may be present during operation and instructions, and (2) precautions for safely operating the equipment or machinery.
Chemical manufacturers	Chemical manufacturers are required to provide downstream users with Safety Data Sheets (SDSs). These summarize information about health hazards, and provide instructions on how to safely handle and use the chemical.
Trade associations, insurance carriers, manufacturers, and government agencies	Some trade associations and insurance carriers publish safety and health information. Some manufacturers, and government agencies such as OSHA, the National Institute for Occupational Safety and Health (NIOSH), issue safety and health warnings and hazard alerts directed toward particular products, work practices, or hazards.
Workplace injury and illness information	Data and reports on occupational injuries, illnesses, and fatalities that have occurred in the workplace provide direct evidence of the presence and seriousness of hazards. Most employers are required to maintain logs and summaries of "recordable" occupational injuries and illnesses and to report incidents to OSHA. Incident investigations can uncover previously undetected hazards and ineffective control measures.
Employee safety and health complaints	Employees have first-hand familiarity with the hazards at their workplace. Any prior or recent complaints about safety and health conditions, whether formal or informal, point to potential safety and health hazards.
Medical surveillance activities, and employee exposure data	These results can alert employers to hazards posed by chemical, physical, and biological agents. Use of aggregated results is important to maintain the confidentiality of employee medical information.
Disaster preparedness scenarios	Conducting a "what-if" analysis of possible natural and man-made disasters can help identify hazards that have a low probability of occurrence, but that may have disastrous consequences. Examples include explosions that could be caused by flammable chemicals or combustible dust, hazards that may be created by strong weather phenomena, or incidents related to a criminal or terrorist act.

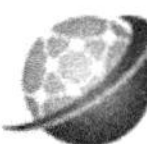

Examples of Hazard Types

Type of Hazard	Source Description and Guidance
Chemical agents	Safety Data Sheets (SDSs) provide a good basis for a developing a list of toxic chemicals in the workplace. When many chemicals are present, hazards of the following types of chemicals should be determined first: chemicals that are (1) volatile; (2) handled or stored in open containers; (3) used in processes where employees are likely to be exposed through inhalation, ingestion, or skin contact; or (4) flammable and stored or used in a manner that poses a fire or explosion hazard.
Biological agents	These include bacteria, viruses, fungi, and other living organisms that can cause acute and chronic infections by entering the body either directly or through breaks in the skin. Sources can include laboratory operations, fermentation processes, or handling of raw food products. They also include exposure to blood or other body fluids or to clients or patients with infectious diseases.
Physical agents	These include excessive levels of ionizing and nonionizing electromagnetic radiation, noise, vibration, illumination, and temperature.
Equipment operation	Ideally, each piece of equipment will be inspected to ensure that all safeguards necessary to protect employees are in place and effective. These include measures to ensure that employees avoid becoming caught in or struck by equipment; burned on hot surfaces; or shocked through contact with energized parts of electric circuits. Important areas of focus for equipment inspection include equipment guarding; the condition of moving parts, parts that support weight, and brakes; and hazards that might arise during maintenance activities
Equipment maintenance	Ideally, the inspection will also include attention to safeguards that ensure that equipment maintenance can be performed safely. This would include such safeguards as de-energizing or otherwise isolating equipment; preventing chemical exposures through appropriate flushing of pumps and other process equipment; releasing stored energy; and use of lockout or tagout to prevent reactivation of equipment during servicing or maintenance.
Fire protection	This part of the inspection would include, for example, making sure that working fire extinguishers are readily available, that flammable liquids and gases are safely handled and stored, and that employees have ready access to emergency exits.
Physical environment	This involves inspecting the facility's walking and working surfaces to identify any trip and fall hazards and ensuring that they are eliminated or controlled.
Work and process flow	The flow of materials and work through an operation can be an important guide to potential hazards. For example, hazards can develop when a product produced at one stage of the process is incompatible with the equipment or practices at the next stage. This could happen in a chemical plant when one piece of equipment produces a hazardous metal catalyst packaged in 55-gallon drums that is then used 5 pounds at a time in another area of the plant. Because of this size difference, employees would need to handle the catalyst manually, causing unnecessary exposures. Producing the catalyst in 5-pound packages would eliminate this hazard.
Work practices	Work practices can be a source of hazards. For example, inappropriate practices for lifting and handling materials can result in back and repetitive motion injuries. When potential hazards are identified, employers can consider whether employees are sufficiently trained to protect themselves. Discussing work practices with employees is particularly important as employees can often identify hazards and solutions based on their day-to-day experience with those practices.

Risk Assessment Matrix: Provides a qualitative method to categorize combinations of indicators and to calculate a risk score.

Example Risk Assessment Matrix

	Severity and Consequences			
Likelihood of Occurrence or exposure	**CATASTROPHIC:** Death or permanent total disability	**CRITICAL:** Disability in excess of 3 months	**MARGINAL:** Minor injury, lost workday	**NEGLIGIBLE:** First aid or minor medical treatment
FREQUENT: Likely to occur repeatedly	HIGH	HIGH	SERIOUS	MEDIUM
PROBABLE: Likely to occur several times	HIGH	HIGH	SERIOUS	MEDIUM
OCCASIONAL: Likely to occur sometime	HIGH	SERIOUS	MEDIUM	LOW
REMOTE: Not Likely to Occur	SERIOUS	MEDIUM	MEDIUM	LOW
IMPROBABLE: Very Unlikely to occur	MEDIUM	LOW	LOW	LOW

Risk Level:

LOW: Risk acceptable or tolerable, remedial action discretionary.
MEDIUM: Take remedial action at appropriate time.
SERIOUS: High priority remedial action.
HIGH: Operation not permissible.

These definitions are provided for illustration purposes and each organization must define these terms as applicable to their process. Adapted from ASSE/ANSI Z-10 2012. These definitions are provided for illustration purposes and each organization must define these terms as applicable to their process.

 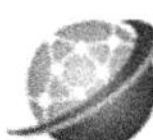

Hazard Prevention and Control

Some ways to prevent and control hazards are:

- Regularly and thoroughly maintain equipment
- Ensure that hazard correction procedures are in place
- Ensure that everyone knows how to use and maintain PPE
- Make sure that everyone understands and follows safe work procedures

Ensure that, when needed, there is a medical program tailored to your facility to help prevent workplace hazards and exposures.

Engineering Controls

The best strategy after elimination or substitution is to control the hazard at its source. Engineering controls do this, unlike other controls that generally focus on the employee exposed to the hazard. The basic concept behind engineering controls is that, to the extent feasible, the work environment and the job itself should be designed to eliminate hazards or reduce exposure to hazards. Engineering controls can be simple in some cases. They are based on the following principles:

- If feasible, design the facility, equipment, or process to remove the hazard or substitute something that is not hazardous.
- If removal is not feasible, enclose the hazard to prevent exposure in normal operations.
- Where complete enclosure is not feasible, establish barriers or local ventilation to reduce exposure to the hazard in normal operations.

Administrative Controls

Administrative controls are measures aimed at reducing employee exposure to hazards. Safe work practices include your company's general workplace rules and other operation-specific rules. These measures may also include additional relief workers, exercise breaks and rotation of workers. These types of controls are normally used in conjunction with other controls that more directly prevent or control exposure to the hazard

Personal Protective Equipment (PPE)
When exposure to hazards cannot be engineered completely out of normal operations or maintenance work, and when safe work practices and other forms of administrative controls cannot provide sufficient additional protection, a supplementary method of control is the use of protective clothing or equipment. This is collectively called personal protective equipment, or PPE. PPE may also be appropriate for controlling hazards while engineering and work practice controls are being installed.

The basic element of any management program for PPE should be an in depth evaluation of the equipment needed to protect against the hazards at the workplace. The evaluation should be used to set a standard operating procedure for personnel, then train employees on the protective limitations of the PPE, and on its proper use and maintenance.

Using PPE requires hazard awareness and training on the part of the user. Employees must be aware that the equipment does not eliminate the hazard. If the equipment fails, exposure will occur. To reduce the possibility of failure, equipment must be properly fitted and maintained in a clean and serviceable condition

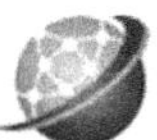

Domain 2 Quiz 1 Questions

1) The **best** protection for laser exposure is an enclosure with
   A) Interlocks.
   B) Glasses.
   C) Signage.
   D) Distance.

2) The **best** solution to eliminate worker exposure to excessive vibrations from tools is:
   A) Provide workers with vibration dampening gloves and wrap the tool in vibration absorbing padding.
   B) Provide tools that are engineered to eliminate operator exposure to vibrations.
   C) Deliver worker safety training to recognize symptoms of vibration related disorders.
   D) Implement work rest cycles and job rotation.

3) An industry had 38 serious incidents including one fatality in the past 15 years. Four incidents involved forklifts. Determine the probability that the next serious accident will involve a forklift.
   A) 13%
   B) A determination is not possible.
   C) 8%
   D) 10.5%

4) A process that seeks to verify documented expectations, typically regulations and policies, by conducting interviews, reviewing records and making first-hand observations is called an:
   A) Site visit.
   B) Management system audit.
   C) Environmental site assessment.
   D) Evaluation assessment and standardization.

5) On a multi-employer steel erection project, the entity that has the overall responsibility for the construction of the project-its planning, quality, and completion is the:

A) Qualified person.
B) Project superintendent.
C) Controlling contractor.
D) Competent person.

6) An environmental Life Cycle Assessment (LCA):

A) Is a stable procedure with few changes over time.
B) Is generally simple and low cost for small firms.
C) Is a systematic process for evaluating environmental impact of products or services.
D) Requires governments to develop enforcement-based environmental regulations.

7) Sustainable development is **best** defined as:

A) A pattern of resource use that aims to meet human needs while preserving the environment so that these needs can be met
B) Meeting the needs of the world's current population without making it impossible for the world's future citizens to meet their needs.
C) Advancement of the principles and goals of sustainable development through partnerships, collaboration, and outreach
D) The interfaces with economics through the social and ecological consequences of economic activity

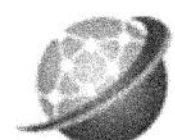

8) While reviewing a bid proposal from a sub-contractor for a lengthy construction job on a large site, the general contractor has proposed several options for developing and complying with safety and health procedures. Which of the following will produce the **most** effective safety and health interface?
   A) The sub-contractor should develop their own procedures and follow them to the letter.
   B) The sub-contractor should use the general contractor's procedures to provide site standardization.
   C) The sub-contractor should follow all the OSHA rules and thus will not need procedures.
   D) The sub-contractor should develop their own procedures with assistance from the general contractor.

9) Considering the waste hierarchy of controls, which is the **least** desirable?
   A) Source reduction/elimination.
   B) Recovery/reuse/recycle.
   C) Waste exchange/energy recovery.
   D) Treatment/destruction/disposal.

10) Generally, system life cycle phases include:
   A) Concept, development, operation and disposal.
   B) Initiation, development, design, evaluation.
   C) Analysis, design, production, disposal.
   D) Concept, sustainment, reliability, disposal.

11) Who is ultimately responsible for hazardous waste from start to finish?
   A) Shipper of the manifested hazardous waste.
   B) Chemical manufactures of the hazardous waste constituents.
   C) Large and small quantity generators of the hazardous waste.
   D) Hazardous waste Treatment and storage and disposal facility.

12) Which legal doctrine is defined by a wrongful act?
   A) Exclusive Remedy.
   B) Gross Negligence.
   C) Tort.
   D) Special Damage.

13) Insurance contracts are unilateral, meaning that only the insurer makes legally enforceable promises in the contract. The insured is not required to pay premiums, but the insurer is required to pay benefits under contract if the insured has paid the premiums and met certain other basic provisions. Which of the following terms represent the general parts of an insurance contract?
   A) Declarations, Definitions, Insuring agreement, Exclusions, Conditions, Endorsements.
   B) Incontestability, Definitions, Conditions, Declarations.
   C) Investigation, Exclusions, Conditions, Privity.
   D) Endorsements, Definitions, Executor, Declaration.

14) An implied warranty is an inference by a wholesaler or manufacturer that merchandise is suitable for a specific function or purpose. The statement of warranty can be made in many ways and could include all of the following **except**
   A) Selling the merchandise for that function.
   B) Marketing that the merchandise will satisfy that function.
   C) Referencing the owner's manual statements that it will accomplish that purpose.
   D) Making the merchandise appear to accomplish the purpose.

15) Which of the following identifies the four mandatory elements for any legal contract?
   A) Consent, legal tender, parties, consideration.
   B) Management, labor, money, contract.
   C) Agreement, consideration, purpose, legal tender.
   D) Agreement, consideration, purpose, competent parties.

16) Three fundamental legal principles that can be used by plaintiffs in product liability cases include
   A) Carelessness, strict legal responsibility, res ipsa loquitar.
   B) Strict liability, express guarantee, implied warranty.
   C) Negligence, strict liability, breach of warranty.
   D) Negligence, strict legal responsibility, tort.

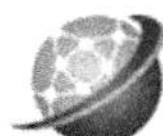

17) Which of the following characteristics of a Product Recall is the **most** important?
   A) Quick response.
   B) Written detailed plan.
   C) Action sheets for each department.
   D) Detailed procedures for notifying authorities and advertising which products are defective.

18) Safety professionals may need to have insurance protection, depending on business status. Out of numerous types of coverage, one specific to safety consultants is professional liability that covers all the following **except:**
   A) Errors and omissions.
   B) Fire damage.
   C) Libel and slander.
   D) Negligence.

19) An agreement or contract in which one party agrees to hold the other free from the responsibility for any liability or damage that might arise out of the transaction involved is called a:
   A) Strict liability.
   B) Hold harmless agreement.
   C) Negligence.
   D) Exclusive remedy.

20) A recreation center has a pool that is not fenced. If a child drowns in the pool, what is the legal doctrine a plaintiff could use in a lawsuit?
   A) Attractive nuisance.
   B) Res ipsa loquitur.
   C) Obvious peril.
   D) Foreseeability.

Domain 2 Quiz 1 Answers

1) Answer A:

Laser radiation of sufficient intensity and exposure time can cause irreversible damage to the skin and eye of man. Control measures shall be devised to reduce the possibility of exposure of the eye and skin to hazardous laser radiation and to other hazards associated with the operation of lasers and laser systems. This applies during normal operation and maintenance by users, as well as by Manufacturers during the manufacture, testing, alignment, servicing, etc. of lasers and laser systems. The four basic categories of controls useful in laser environments are engineering controls, personal protective equipment, administrative and procedural controls, and special controls. (ANSI Z-136.1). There are some uses of Class IIIB and IV Class IV lasers where the entire beam path may be totally enclosed, other uses where the beam path is confined by design to significantly limit access and yet other uses where the beam path is totally open. In each case, the controls required will vary as follows:

- ENCLOSED (TOTAL) BEAM PATH: Perhaps the most common form of a Class I laser system is a high power laser that has been totally enclosed (embedded) inside a protective enclosure equipped with appropriate interlocks and/or labels on all removable panels or access doors. Beam access is prevented, therefore, during operation and maintenance. Such a completely enclosed system, if properly labeled and properly safeguarded with a protective housing interlocks (and all other applicable engineering controls), will fulfill all requirements for a Class I laser and may be operated in the enclosed manner WITH NO ADDITIONAL CONTROLS for the operator. It should be noted that during periods of service or maintenance, controls appropriate to the class of the embedded laser may be required (perhaps on a temporary basis) when the beam enclosures are removed and beam access is possible. Beam access during maintenance or service procedures will not alter the Class I status of the laser during operation.
- LIMITED OPEN BEAM PATH: It is becoming quite commonplace, particularly with some industrial materials processing lasers, to have an enclosure that surrounds the area around the laser focusing optics and encloses the immediate area of the workstation almost completely. Often, a computer controlled positioning table is located within this enclosure; there is often a gap of less than one-quarter of an inch between the bottom of the enclosure and the top of the material to be laser processed. Such a design provides the needed mobility relative to the stationary laser. Such a system would not meet, perhaps, the stringent "human

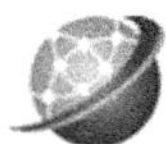

access" requirements of the Federal Laser Product Performance Standard (FLPPS) for a Class I laser, but the real laser hazards are well confined. Such a design provides what can be called a limited open beam path. In this situation, the ANSI Z-136.1 standard recommends that the Laser Safety Officer (LSO) shall effect a laser hazard analysis and establish the extent of the Nominal Hazard Zone (NHZ). In many system designs, (such as described above), the NHZ will be extremely limited and procedural controls (rather than elaborate engineering controls) will be sufficient. Such an installation will require a detailed standard operating procedure (SOP). Training is also needed for the system operator commensurate with the class of the embedded laser. Protective equipment (eye protection, temporary barriers, clothing and/or gloves, respirators ...etc) would be recommended, for example, only if the hazard analysis indicated a need or if the SOP required periods of beam access such as during setup or infrequent maintenance activities. Temporary protective measures for service is handled in a manner similar to service of any embedded Class IV laser.

- TOTALLY UNENCLOSED BEAM PATH: There are several specific applications areas where high power (Class IIIB and Class IV) lasers are used in an unenclosed beam condition. This would include for example, open industrial processing systems (often incorporating robotic delivery), laser research laboratory installations, surgical installations...etc. Such laser uses will require that a complete hazard analysis and NHZ assessment be effected by the LSO. Then, the controls implemented will reflect the magnitude and extent of hazards associated with the accessible beam.

2) Answer B:

The best solution is to use a tool that is has engineered safety through the design phase. Eliminating the vibration transferred from the tool to the operator. (NIOSH, 1997) Examples of engineering controls for ergonomics include:

- Changing the way materials, parts, and prod-ucts can be transported-for example, using mechanical assist devices to relieve heavy load lifting and carrying tasks or using han-dles or slotted hand holes in packages requir-ing manual handling
- Changing the process or product to reduce worker exposures to risk factors; examples include maintaining the fit of plastic molds to reduce the need for manual removal of flash-ing, or using easy-connect electrical termi-nals to reduce manual forces
- Modifying containers and parts presentation, such as height-adjustable

material bins

- Changing workstation layout, which might include using height-adjustable workbenches or locating tools and materials within short reaching distances
- Changing the way parts, tools, and materials are to be manipulated; examples include us-ing fixtures (clamps, vise-grips, etc.) to hold work pieces to relieve the need for awkward hand and arm positions or suspending tools to reduce weight and allow easier access
- Changing tool designs-for example, pistol handle grips for knives to reduce wrist bend-ing postures required by straight-handle knives or squeeze-grip-actuated screwdrivers to replace finger-trigger-actuated screwdrivers
- Changes in materials and fasteners (for exam-ple, lighter-weight packaging materials to re-duce lifting loads)

3) Answer D:

Probability is the number of fork truck accidents divided by the number of total accidents.

$$P = \frac{4}{38} = 0.105 = 10.5\%$$

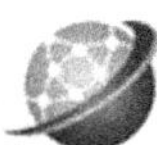

4) Answer B:

This is the definition of an environmental audit, sometimes called a compliance audit. An environmental site assessment is a process that seeks to characterize a physical property or operation from an environmental view with an overall objective of understanding site-specific conditions. Information is collected through interviews, record reviews and first-hand observations. It may also involve testing environmental media and facility characteristics. These definitions are not used consistently throughout the profession, so ensure you are clear about specified definitions with all parties engaged in operations.

5) Answer C:

In the OSHA Steel Erection Standard, the controlling contractor has specific responsibilities. Controlling contractor means a prime contractor, general contractor, construction manager or any other legal entity that has the overall responsibility for the construction of the project-it's planning, quality, and completion. _The standard placed these duties on the controlling contractor because, as the contractor with general supervisory authority over the worksite, it is in the best position to comply with them. None of these provisions require the controlling contractor to direct the individual employees of a subcontractor or supplier. The extent of the measures that a controlling employer must implement to satisfy this duty of reasonable care is less than what is required of an employer with respect to protecting its own employees. This means that the controlling employer is not normally required to inspect for hazards as frequently or to have the same level of knowledge of the applicable standards or of trade expertise as the employer it has hired.

6) Answer C:

As a means of relieving government of costly enforcement based environmental regulations, some countries are establishing product-oriented incentives that are intended to yield environmental benefits. The basis for evaluating such incentives is the province of Life Cycle Assessment (LCA). ISO 14040, the Life Cycle Assessment Guideline, defines LCA as a systematic set of procedures for compiling and examining the inputs and outputs of materials and energy and the associated environmental impacts directly attributable to the functioning of a product or service system throughout its life cycle.

7) Answer B:

Sustainable development has been defined by the United Nations World Commission on Environment and Development as meeting the needs of the world's current population without making it impossible for the world's future citizens to meet their needs. The global nature of this definition often makes implementation challenging within business organizations. Those businesses that are ready to make sustainable development operational begin by transforming principles, behaviors, and practices involved in their basic internal workings. Those base principles and behaviors have to do with: Transparency in business objectives and practices; Governance practices including business environmental ethics; Social responsibility programs including community, workforce, and other involved stakeholders Environmental health and safety processes based on continuous improvement. Sustainable development, like EMS, requires the development of indicators (leading or lagging), and metrics against them to measure and verify improvements in the categories mentioned. These measures go together with the concept of the triple bottom line, under which companies are evaluated by stakeholders not only on financial performance, but also on environmental and social performance. As an extension of this, many businesses now include environmental and social performance in their annual reporting to shareholders. Environmental aspects that readily lend themselves to the development of metrics include: Consideration of residuals (e.g., air emissions, waste water, and solid and hazardous waste); Energy and material inputs and outputs associated with a process; Life-cycle environmental costs of the product or service produced.

8) Answer D:

The current opinion is that the sub-contractors should develop their own procedures with help from the general contractor. This method will assure maximum standardization and flexibility while assuring effective accident prevention programs. This interface not only is effective it helps each party to understand the concerns of each other and allows both sides to develop better programs. Blind adherence to the general contractors program usually does not work and just causes problems. For example, the requirement of a general to use a particular type of fall protection or hardhat or eye protection may cause hardship for the sub-contractor. On the other hand the use of a standardized general class of fall protection, or head protection etc. is going to be required by the general, so some collaboration will be required. That is, the sub probably cannot follow your procedures to the letter, so you both might as well establish some rules everyone can live with.

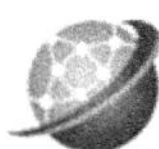

9) Answer D:

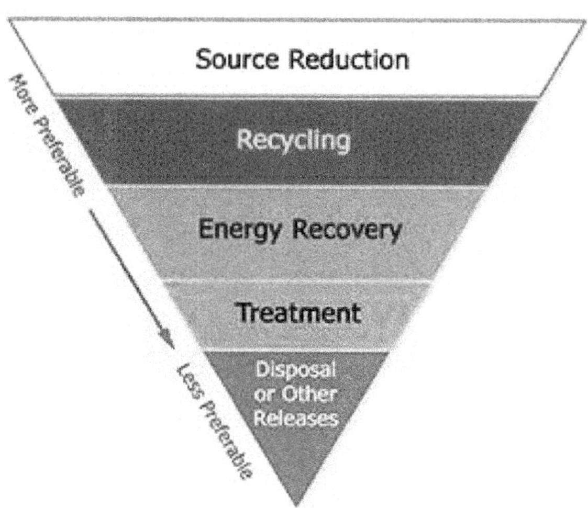

EPA developed the non-hazardous materials and waste management hierarchy in recognition that no single waste management approach is suitable for managing all materials and waste streams in all circumstances. The hierarchy ranks the various management strategies from most to least environmentally preferred. The hierarchy places emphasis on reducing, reusing, and recycling as key to sustainable materials management.

10) Answer A:

According to Haight (2012), there are **four major phases of development in a system life cycle: (1) concept, (2) system development, (3) production and deployment, and (4) sustainment and disposal**. Each phase includes safety engineering tasks that result in a formal decision about proceeding to the next phase. A system-safety management plan should be developed during the concept phase in order to design safety into the system and maintain it throughout the system's life. Incorporating system safety early in development increases the probability that hazards can be addressed more economically and with greater efficiency. A formal decision earmarks the acceptance of risks) to that point of development or operation.

System safety is a comprehensive approach for integrating safety as part of the design-and implementing requirements throughout other phases-in the life cycle of a system, product, process, or facility. The primary function of system safety is to identify and control hazards in each phase of the life cycle, from concept through decommissioning and disposal. In system development, anticipating potential hazards and conditions is a key aspect of safety engineering work. It is a challenge to anticipate the hazards of a system before it is developed; however, safety engineering activities designed into each phase promote a systematic process of anticipating and identifying hazards as the system is developed. According to Brauer (1990), "System safety is ... the systematic, forward-looking identification and control of hazards ...." Safety engineers assess the existing and potential conditions that could affect a system.

11) Answer C:
In keeping with the cradle-to-grave concept, waste continues to be the property of the generator. Any discrepancies in the waste shipment must be reported to EPA. The current hazardous waste manifest system is a set of forms, reports, and procedures designed to seamlessly track hazardous waste from the time it leaves the generator facility where it was produced, until it reaches the off-site waste management facility that will store, treat, or dispose of the hazardous waste. The system allows the waste generator to verify that its waste has been properly delivered, and that no waste has been lost or unaccounted for in the process. The current Hazardous Waste Manifest is a joint undertaking by EPA and the Department of Transportation (DOT). EPA is responsible for regulating hazardous waste under a Federal statute known as the Resource Conservation and Recovery Act (RCRA). This Act requires that all hazardous waste shipped off-site be tracked from **"cradle-to-grave"** using a manifest that provides information about the generator of the waste, the facility that will receive the waste, a description and quantity of the waste (including the number and type of containers), and how the waste will be routed to the receiving facility. Because hazardous waste is also regulated by the DOT under its hazardous materials laws, the Manifest was developed to meet both EPA's requirements for a manifest, and DOT's requirements for "shipping papers."

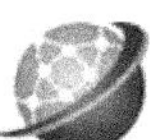

Conditionally Exempt Small Quantity Generator (CESQG)

- Generated
  - Less than 100 kg/mo of any hazardous waste
  - Less than 1 kg/mo of P-listed (acutely hazardous) waste
  - Less than 100 kg/mo of cleanup waste
- Accumulated
  - Less than 1,000 kg of any hazardous waste
  - Less than 1 kg of P-listed (acutely hazardous) waste
  - Less than 100 kg of cleanup waste

Small Quantity Generator (SQG)

- Generated:
  - 100 and 1,000 kg per month of hazardous waste
  - No more than 1 kg of acutely hazardous waste
- Have limitations on accumulation as follows:
  - Accumulation time without permit is less than or equal to 180 days.
  - Accumulation quantity is limited to 6,000 kg
  - Accumulation is allowed in tanks or containers only

Large Quantity Generator (LQG)

- Is subject to full Subtitle C regulation
- <u>Generates more than SQG and CESQG</u>
  - More than 1,000 kg/mo of any hazardous waste
  - More than 1 kg/mo of acutely hazardous waste
- Accumulates more than SQG and CESQG
  - More than 6,000 kg of hazardous waste
  - More than 1 kg of acutely hazardous waste
  - More than 100 kg of contaminated soil, waste, or debris

12) Answer C:

A wrongful act, or failure to exercise due care, for which civil legal action can result is the definition of ***Tort.*** The concept that a producer of a product is liable for injuries due to defects, without the necessity for plaintiff to show negligence or fault is known as **Strict Liability**. **Exclusive Remedy:** State workers' compensation statutes gave employees a definite remedy for injuries and diseases arising out of or suffered in the course of their employment. In exchange for a definite recovery, the workers' compensation remedy is exclusive, that is, with just a few exceptions, a worker's right of recovery against the employer is limited to the benefits provided by the workers' compensation law. The employee may not sue in tort. A legal doctrine that an employer who is normally immune from tort actions by employees because of workers' compensation laws may be held liable for additional damages as a party who has committed a wrongful or negligent act beyond its role as employer.Example: An employee of an aerosol shaving cream manufacturer is injured by an exploding can while handling stock. The manufacturer is liable to the employee under workers' compensation laws, but it may also be held responsible for manufacturing a defective can. The employee then may choose to bring a civil suit, where the potential recovery is greater than the statutory remedy of workers' compensation. **Special Damages:** Special damages are one actually sustained, rather than implied by law. They are either added to general damages arising from an act injurious in itself; such as when some particular loss arises from the uttering of slanderous words, actionable in themselves; or are such as arise from an act not actionable in itself, but injurious only in its consequences; such as when the words become actionable only by reason of special damage ensuing. To constitute special damage, the legal and natural consequence must arise from the tort - not from a mere wrongful act of a third person or a remote consequence. The exercise of reasonable care in the handling and preservation of a product in their possession so that it will not later cause injury to a user is the definition of *"Responsibility for Handling"*. A person may be held liable for actions that result in injury or damage only when he was able to foresee dangers and risks that could be reasonably anticipated is the definition of ***"Foreseeability"***.

13) Answer A:

The parts of an insurance contract include:

- Declarations - identify who is an insured, insured's address, insuring company, what risks or property are covered, policy limits (amount of insurance), any applicable deductibles, policy period and premium amount. These are usually provided on a form that is completed by the insurer based on the insured's application and attached on top of or inserted within the first few pages of a standard policy form.
- Definitions - define important terms used in policy language.
- Insuring agreement - describes the covered perils, or risks assumed, or nature of coverage, or makes some reference to the contractual agreement between insurer and insured. It summarizes the major promises of the insurance company, as well as stating what is covered.

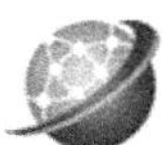

- Exclusions – negates coverage from Insuring Agreement by describing property, perils, hazards or losses arising from specific causes which are **not** covered by the policy.
- Conditions - provisions, rules of conduct, duties and obligations required for coverage. If policy conditions are not met, the insurer can deny the claim.
- Endorsements - additional forms attached to the policy form that modify it in some way, either unconditionally or upon existence of some condition. Endorsements can make policies difficult to read for non-lawyers; they may modify or delete clauses located several pages earlier in the standard insuring agreement, or even modify each other. Because it is very risky to allow non-lawyer underwriters to directly rewrite core policy language with word processors. Insurers usually direct underwriters to modify standard forms by attaching endorsements preapproved by counsel for various common modifications.

14) Answer D:

Implied warranty is the implication by a dealer that the product will serve a specific purpose. The implication must be made by

- Placing it on sale for that purpose
- Advertising it for that purpose
- Indicating in books or manuals that it will operate in a manner that could reasonably be interpreted as being suitable for that purpose

15) Answer D:

A legal contract must have four parts:

- Agreement
- Consideration
- Purpose
- Competent parties

16) Answer C:

The three basic legal principles that can be used in most states are:

- Negligence, which tests the conduct of the defendant
- Strict liability and implied warranty, which test product quality
- Express warranty and misrepresentation, which test product performance against the manufacturer/seller's representations. This may be referred to as Breach of Warranty.

17) Answer B:
The single most important part of a successful product recall is the establishment of a detailed written plan that outlines individual and company responsibilities and actions. This "Emergency Action Plan" must encompass all aspects of a recall and could include items such as communication of a warning if necessary; details of the hazard; instructions for continued usage or return; removal and modification of existing products from inventory; compensation for injury; investigation of the causes of error, lack of warning, or design etc.

18) Answer B:
Safety Consultants Professional Liability covers errors and omissions, libel and slander, negligence, oral and written publication of information that causes damage and infringement upon copyrighted materials. Safety Consultants Commercial General Liability covers bodily injury/property damage, fire damage and medical expenses.

19) Answer B:

A ***Hold Harmless (Indemnity) Agreement*** is used between two parties to establish that the indemnitee is protected from any unforeseen liabilities, losses, claims or damages during their involvement in an activity. A Hold Harmless Agreement is developed to prevent law suits by assigning liability in a contract. Hold harmless means that if there is a problem and a suit later, one party shields or "holds harmless" the other. A hold harmless clause is a statement in a legal contract stating that an individual or organization is not liable for any injuries or damages caused to the individual signing the contract. An individual may be asked to sign a hold harmless agreement when undertaking an activity that involves risk for which the enabling entity does not want to be legally or financially responsible. **Strict liability** is the concept whereby the plaintiff need not show negligence or fault to prove liability. **Negligence** is the failure to exercise a reasonable amount of care or to carry out a legal duty so that injury or property damage occurs to another. An example would be you were a landlord and did not provide adequate security and the renter was robbed. **Exclusive Remedy:** State workers' compensation statutes gave employees a definite remedy for injuries and diseases arising out of or suffered in the course of their employment. In exchange for a definite recovery, the workers' compensation remedy is exclusive, that is, with just a few exceptions, a worker's right of recovery against the employer is limited to the benefits provided by the workers' compensation law. The employee may not sue in tort.

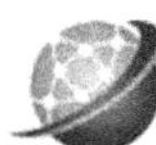

20) Answer A:

The **attractive nuisance** doctrine applies to the law of torts, in the United States. It states that a landowner may be held liable for injuries to children trespassing on the land if the injury is caused by an object on the land that is likely to attract children. **Tort** is a wrongful act or a failure to exercise due care that results in damage or injury in the broadest sense. A manufacturer or distributor would not have to label a large blade hunting knife because the product involves an **obvious peril**, sometimes called an obvious hazard that is well known to the public. The term **res ipsa loquitur** (the thing speaks for itself) is involved in accidents where the damage producing agent was under the sole control of the defendant and the accident would not have happened if the defendant would have exercised proper control. **Foreseeability** involves the liability for actions that a normal person would have known to exist and would have taken precautions to prevent.

Domain 2 Quiz 2 Questions

1) Any action which reduces losses incurred, by definition, is
   A) Loss control.
   B) Loss transfer.
   C) Risk management.
   D) Loss reduction.

2) Which of the following is **most** crucial in conducting a successful hazard and operability study?
   A) Numerous labor and management representatives knowledgeable of safety procedures.
   B) A study director familiar with the process being considered.
   C) A conversant process safety engineer familiar with process safety regulations.
   D) Multiple subject matter experts knowledgeable about the process being studied.

3) Common substance abuse testing policies include:
   A) Annual, pre-hire screening, random, post incident.
   B) Post-incident, suspicion, random, monthly.
   C) Pre-employment, random, reasonable suspicion, post-incident.
   D) Pre-hire, monthly, random, post-incident.

4) What is the term for the ratio of risk exposure to venture or project cost?
   A) Expenditure ratio.
   B) Loss/profit ratio.
   C) Risk exposure ratio.
   D) Threat ratio.

5) The stages in the risk analysis and management of a project include all of the following **except**
   A) Identification.
   B) Estimation.
   C) Response.
   D) Intervention.

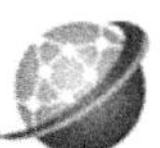

6) Risk assessment should be carried out by a(an):
   A) Supervisor.
   B) Enforcement officer.
   C) Competent person.
   D) Safety representative.

7) A method used to reduce risk is known as a:
   A) Hazard.
   B) Control measure.
   C) Hazard report.
   D) Safety analysis.

8) An example of a human factor that could result in an accident is:
   A) High noise levels.
   B) A dusty workplace.
   C) Inexperience.
   D) Poor lighting.

9) Risk assessment must be carried out in:
   A) All workplaces.
   B) Some workplaces.
   C) Only large workplaces.
   D) Only high-risk workplaces.

10) Which one of the following procedures employs deductive analysis?
   A) Failure Mode and Effect Analysis (FMEA).
   B) Fault Tree Analysis (FTA).
   C) Preliminary Hazard Analysis (PHA).
   D) Operational Hazard Analysis (OHA).

11) Which is the **best** definition of hazard?
   A) A condition, set of circumstances, or inherent property that can cause injury, illness, or death.
   B) An event in which a work related injury or illness or fatality occurred or could have occurred
   C) A set of interrelated elements that establish and support occupational safety and health objectives.
   D) An estimate of the combination of the likelihood of an occurrence of a hazardous event or exposure, and the severity of the injury.

12) Risk is a combination of:
   A) Frequency of episodes of an adverse event and probability of occurrence of the adverse event.
   B) Probability that an adverse event will occur and consequences of the adverse event.
   C) Probability that a hazardous condition exists and consequences of the hazard.
   D) Exposure and consequences to a particular hazard.

13) Which of the following is **least important** when performing a risk assessment to estimate, evaluate, and reduce risks associated with machining tools?
   A) Probability of occurrence.
   B) Severity of harm.
   C) Cost benefit ratio of risk reduction options.
   D) Exposure to hazard.

14) Which of the following is considered a direct cost when defining hidden costs of an accident?
   A) Time lost from work by injured.
   B) Time lost by fellow workers.
   C) Payment and benefits for lost time.
   D) Loss of production.

15) Which of the following **best** describes a simplified semi-qualitative method of risk assessment that is between qualitative process hazard analysis and a traditional, expensive quantitative risk analysis?
   A) Hazard Operability Study.
   B) Layer of Protection Analysis.
   C) Failure Modes Effects Analysis.
   D) What-If /Checklist Study.

16) Which of the following is **not** considered loss reduction?
   A) Providing a CPR/first aid certified individual on every work team.
   B) Installing a modernized fire suppression system.
   C) Doing emergency planning (what if) scenarios.
   D) Storing back up files at an offsite location.

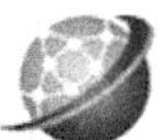

17) What is the **primary** function of a loss control system?
   A) Assess risk, establish effective risk control measures, and elimination of risk.
   B) Establish effective risk control measures for hazardous conditions, establish effective control measures, elimination of risk.
   C) Identify hazardous conditions, assess their risks, and establish effective risk control measures.
   D) Assure compliance with applicable regulatory requirements and eliminate residual risk.

18) Accepted probabilistic risk assessment methodology used for assessing workplace system failures is called ______ analysis.
   A) Environmental.
   B) Fault tree.
   C) Job safety.
   D) Safety and health.

19) When implementing a JSA program, which of the following is the **first** item to be analyzed?
   A) Order of Jobs according to product flow moving through each department.
   B) Jobs generating most complaints from supervisors.
   C) Jobs contributing to highest incident rates.
   D) Jobs exposing most workers.

20) The **best** description for a management system's use of the accident cycle is:
   A) Reactive.
   B) Proactive.
   C) Employee driven.
   D) Preventative.

Domain 2 Quiz 2 Answers

1) Answer D:

Loss reduction means any **action** which reduces the losses incurred. The reduction may be by decrease of the physical destruction (as by reducing the amount of material burned or the number of persons injured) or by reducing the operational loss from a given amount of destruction (as having standby equipment or more effective medical care for the injured). It includes the concepts of loss prevention and control as well as the concept of risk avoidance—the refusal to accept a given risk. Planning actions are not generally considered part of loss reduction. The four steps required in an effective loss control program are problem identification, selection of corrective measures, implementation and feedback and control.

2) Answer D:

As referenced in by the Center for Chemical Process Safety *Guidelines for Hazard Evaluation Procedures,* 2nd Edition, subject matter experts familiar with the process and sections of the process being studied are essential. A process hazard analysis leader familiar with the analytical method is important, but it is not essential for the study leader to be personally familiar with the actual process being studied.

3) Answer C:

Whether the substance abuse occurs at home or at work, employees who abuse alcohol and drugs (including illegal drugs, prescription drugs, and over-the-counter drugs) can create significant issues for both employers and other employees. Employees who abuse drugs have been shown to have lower job performance, reduced productivity, and greater absenteeism, not to mention higher medical and workers' compensation costs. Substance abuse testing policies generally involve:

- Pre-employment
- Reasonable suspicion
- Post-incident
- Random
- Conditions for return to work and termination

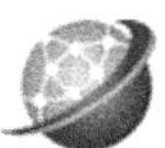

An Employee Assistance Program (EAP) is a voluntary, confidential program that helps employees (including management) work through various life challenges that may adversely affect job performance, health, and personal well-being to optimize an organization's success. EAP services include assessments, counseling, and referrals for additional services to employees with personal and/or work-related concerns, such as stress, financial issues, legal issues, family problems, office conflicts, and alcohol and substance use disorders. EAPs also often work with management and supervisors providing advanced planning for situations, such as organizational changes, legal considerations, emergency planning, and response to unique traumatic events. EAPs can reap benefits for organizations, employees, families, and communities by:

- Improving productivity and employee engagement;
- Improving employees' and dependents' abilities to successfully respond to challenges;
- Developing employee and manager competencies in managing workplace stress;
- Reducing workplace absenteeism and unplanned absences;
- Supporting employees and managers during workforce restructuring, reduction-in-forces, or other workforce change events;
- Reducing workplace accidents;
- Reducing the likelihood of workplace violence or other safety risks;
- Supporting disaster and emergency preparedness;
- Managing the effect of disruptive incidents, such as workplace, injury, or other crises;
- Facilitating safe, timely, and effective return-to-work for employees short-term and extended absences;
- Reducing healthcare costs associated with stress, depression, and other mental health issues; and
- Reducing employee turnover and related replacement costs.

4) Answer C:
Risk exposure ratio is the ratio of the risk exposure to the project cost. Risk exposure is a quantified loss potential of business. Risk exposure is usually calculated by multiplying the probability of an incident occurring by its potential losses. When considering loss probability, businesses usually divide risk into two categories: pure risk and speculative risk. Pure risks are categories of risk that are beyond anyone's control, such as natural disasters or untimely death. Speculative risks can be taken on voluntarily. Types of speculative risk include financial investments or any activities that will result in either a profit or a loss for the business. Speculative risks carry an uncertain outcome. Potential losses incurred by speculative risks could stem from business liability issues, property loss, property damage, strained customer relations and increased overhead expenses. To calculate risk exposure, variables are determined to calculate the probability of the risk occurring. These are then multiplied by the total potential loss of the risk. To determine the variables, organizations must know the total loss in dollars that might occur, as well as a percentage depicting the probability of the risk occurring. The objective of the risk exposure calculation is to determine the overall level of risk that the organization can tolerate for the given situation, based on the benefits and costs involved. The level of risk an organization is prepared to accept is called its risk appetite.

5) Answer D:
There are five stages in risk analysis and management:

1). identification
2). estimation
3). evaluation
4). response
5). monitoring

Identification techniques include individual consultation and group discussion. Individual consultations are one-on-one meetings are arranged as a preliminary exercise to initially identify the risks. This process involves key participants in the project in question. The purpose of this stage is to allow the interviewee to contemplate what he/she thinks are the main risks attached to either, the project as a whole, or as individual stages of the project or both. As the participants are from different disciplines, their viewpoints about the project are influenced by the specialized nature of their field. Group discussion is a process by which potential sources of risk are identified with a clear set of rules and a timetable. This technique should be carried out with the project team. One person should

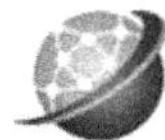

be the coordinator who chairs the meetings. The discussion process should have two distinct stages, a creative stage and an assessment stage. The creative stage permits any one member of the team, one at a time, to 'throw' in potential risks or sources of risk. Individual team members are not restricted to their own knowledge domain and outlandish ideas are encouraged. The assessment stage then follows. Estimation includes interviewing and brain-storming with personal and corporate experience. The analysis, and/or estimation, stage is more extensive in nature than in the identification stage. All the ideas are analyzed individually and a final draft of the risks is assembled. The idea of the analysis stage is to categorize or rank the risks by using the one-on-one situation in interviewing, or the group discussions from brain-storming. Therefore, the end result from this stage is to prioritize the risks so as to know which of them are to be forwarded to the quantitative analysis. At this point, this threshold level or cut-off point must also be decided. The notion being the risks below this level, and thus those not to be analyzed quantitatively, are covered by project contingent reserves. The ones above would not be, hence requiring further analysis.

Personal and Corporate experience. If there are employees with experience, then this property should be utilized. Experience enables the main risks in a project to be identified. Obviously, one looks at the more senior officers to excel in this department. However, there is always a chance that certain risks never encountered before are overlooked. If the project is not equivalent to a previous project, then the policies of the company, or engineering judgment decides on a contingency percentage. Factors of safety are used extensively in the construction industry and is based on this method. Response strategies include:

Risk Avoidance

Avoiding risk can be as simple as a contractor not placing a bid or even the owner not proceeding with project funding. Other ways are: tendering at a very high bid, placing conditions on the bid and not bidding on the high-risk portion of the contract.

Risk Transfer

Risk transfer can take two basic forms:

The property or activity responsible for the risk may be transferred, e.g. hire a subcontractor to work on a hazardous process, and

The property or activity may be retained, but the financial risk transferred, e.g. insurance or client takes the costs of risk by contract

Risk Retention
This is the method of responding to risks by the body who controls them. The risks, foreseen or unforeseen, are controlled and financed by the company or contractor that is fulfilling the terms of contract. There are two retention methods, active and passive. Active retention, sometimes referred to as self-insurance, is a deliberate management strategy after a conscious evaluation of the possible losses and costs of alternative ways of handling risks. Passive retention, on the other hand, (sometimes called non-insurance) occurs through neglect, ignorance or absence of decision, e.g. a risk has not been identified and responding to the consequences of that risk must be borne by the contractor performing the work.

Risk Reduction
Loss prevention is one of the ways of risk reduction. Loss prevention can be classified into four basic categories:
Preconditions for a loss, i.e. faults in the premises, e.g. badly insulated wire,
Prevention of loss; devices designed to prevent preconditions for loss, e.g. cut-off switches
Early discovery of loss producing events, e.g. sprinkler system
Limitation of loss, e.g. fire doors, compartmentalization.

6) Answer C:

The term "Competent Person" is used in many OSHA standards and documents. An OSHA "competent person" is defined as "one who is capable of identifying existing and predictable hazards in the surroundings or working conditions which are unsanitary, hazardous, or dangerous to employees, and who has authorization to take prompt corrective measures to eliminate them" 29 CFR 1926.32(f). By way of training and/or experience, a competent person is knowledgeable of applicable standards, is capable of identifying workplace hazards relating to the specific operation, and has the authority to correct them. Some standards add additional specific requirements which must be met by the competent person. Another definition is a person with the appropriate combination of skill, knowledge, qualifications and experience should conduct the risk assessment.

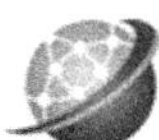

7) Answer B:

Risk management is the identification, assessment, and prioritization of risks (defined in ISO 31000 as *the effect of uncertainty on objectives*) followed by coordinated and economical application of resources to minimize, monitor, and control the probability and/or impact of unfortunate events or to maximize the realization of opportunities. Once risks have been identified and assessed, all techniques to manage the risk fall into one or more of these control measures:

- Avoidance (eliminate, withdraw from or not become involved)
- Reduction (optimize – mitigate)
- Sharing (transfer – outsource or insure)
- Retention (accept and budget)

Ideal use of these strategies may not be possible. Some of them may involve trade-offs that are not acceptable to the organization or person making the risk management decisions.

8) Answer C:

Not understanding properly how something works or an error in diagnosis or planning can be due to inexperience. Increasing the knowledge and experience of employees will result in greater competence to reduce accidents.

9) Answer A:

According to ANSI/ASSE/ISO 31000 (Z690.2-2011) *Risk Management Principles and Guidelines* organizations of all types and sizes face internal and external factors and influences that make it uncertain whether and when they will achieve their objectives. The effect this uncertainty has on an organization's objectives is "risk". All activities of an organization involve risk. Organizations manage risk by identifying it, analyzing it and then evaluating whether the risk should be modified by risk treatment in order to satisfy their risk criteria. Throughout this process, they communicate and consult with stakeholders and monitor and review the risk and the controls that are modifying the risk in order to ensure that no further risk treatment is required. This standard describes this systematic and logical process in detail.

10) Answer B:

Deductive analysis involves reasoning from the general to the specific. Of the choices listed only Fault Tree Analysis involves this technique.

11) Answer A:
Hazard: A condition, set of circumstances, or inherent property that can cause injury, illness, or death.
Incident: An event in which a work related injury or illness or fatality occurred or could have occurred
Occupational Health and Safety Management System (OHSMS): A set of interrelated elements that establish and support occupational safety and health objectives.
Risk: An estimate of the combination of the likelihood of an occurrence of a hazardous event or exposure, and the severity of the injury.

12) Answer B:
Risk is defined as the probability that a substance or situation will produce harm under specified conditions. Risk is a combination of two factors:
1) The probability that an adverse event will occur and
2) The consequences of the adverse event.
Risk encompasses impacts on public health and environment, and arises from exposure and hazard. Risk does not exist if exposure to a harmful substance or situation does not or will not occur. Hazard is determined by whether a particular substance or situation has the potential to cause harmful effects. Risk is the probability of a specific outcome, generally adverse, given a particular set of conditions.

13) Answer C:
Risk assessment was introduced and specifically addressed by the American National Standards Institute in ANSI B11.TR3:2000 entitled *Risk assessment and risk reduction–A guide to estimate, evaluate, and reduce risks associated with machine tools*. The ANSI B11.TR3 explored three major premises of risks:

- probability of occurrence—very likely, likely, unlikely, or remote
- severity of harm—catastrophic, serious, moderate, or minor
- exposure to hazard—frequency and duration, extent of exposure, or number of people exposed

ANSI B11.TR3 explains that zero risk does not exist and is therefore unattainable. Some amount of residual risk remains even after the application of machine safeguarding. Cost benefit is not part of a Risk Assessment. In essence, the common primary objective in both ANSI B11.TR3 and ANSI B11-2008 is that reasonably foreseeable hazards must be identified and dealt with. Both standards contain scoring/rating systems to establish various risk reduction categories. The European Machinery Standard EN1050 (now ISO 14121) follows the same general format and addresses risk assessment in the same

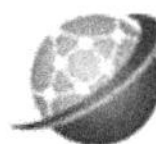

manner. However, it utilizes terms and phrases which are common to European standards.

14) Answer C:
The direct costs are medical and compensation. The indirect or hidden costs are: time lost from work by the injured, loss in earning power, economic loss to the injured family, lost time by fellow workers, loss of efficiency due to break-up of crew, lost time by supervision, cost of breaking in a new worker, damage to tools and equipment, time damaged equipment is out of service, spoiled work, loss of production, spoilage, failure to fill orders, overhead costs and miscellaneous.

15) Answer B:
According to “Layers of Protection Analysis: Simplified Process Risk Assessment,” Center for Chemical Process Safety, American Institute of Chemical Engineers (2001), layers of protection analysis (LOPA) is a powerful analytical tool for assessing the adequacy of protection layers used to mitigate process risk. LOPA builds upon well-known process hazards analysis techniques, applying semi-quantitative measures to the evaluation of the frequency of potential incidents and the probability of failure of the protection layers. Beginning with an identified accident scenario, LOPA uses simplifying rules to evaluate initiating event frequency, independent layers of protection, and consequences to provide an order-of-magnitude estimate of risk. LOPA has also proven an excellent approach for determining the safety integrity level necessary for an instrumented safety system, an approach endorsed in instrument standards, such as ISA S84 and IEC 61511.

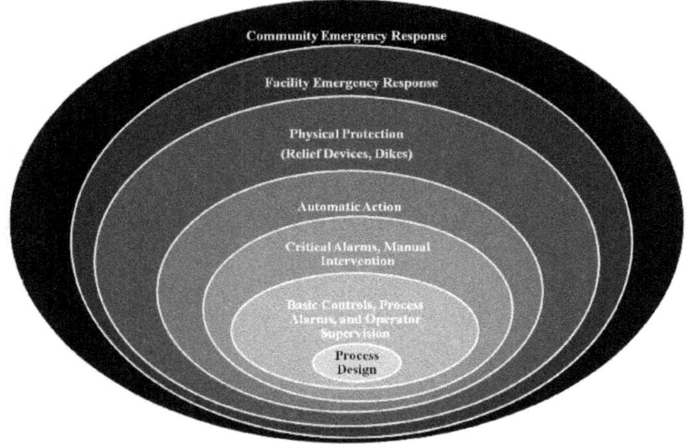

16) Answer D:
Storing back up files at an offsite location would be considered loss prevention and not loss reduction. Other examples of loss prevention are replacing physical guards on saws, installing GFCIs or performing HAZCOM training. An example of loss reduction would be to equip and train a fire brigade. Loss reduction has several approaches. Risk management control procedures emphasize safety management. The human approach believes the safety attitudes of individuals determine the safety precautions they take. The engineering approach places emphasis on physical features of the workplace as a potential cause of injuries. Another approach is reducing operational loss from a given amount of destruction (e.g. by having stand-by equipment or more effective medical care for the injured).

17) Answer C:
As described in *Assurance Technologies*, a loss control system must be able to identify the hazardous conditions as well as understand the real risks associated with those hazardous conditions. A loss control system is incomplete if it solely identifies hazardous conditions and does not take action to understand the risks. Therefore, the actions taken are relative to the risks associated with the hazardous conditions.

18) Answer B:
Fault tree analysis is a commonly used method for assessing system reliability. It starts with a top-level fault and works down, identifying the events that make that top event occur and using component probabilities to calculate ultimate probability the event may occur. A system is analyzed in the context of its work environment and actual operation to find all credible ways in which the system can fail.

19) Answer C:
In the NSC *Accident Prevention Manual for Business and Industry: Administration and Programs,* 12th Edition, the jobs selected for job safety analyses should not be selected at random. The order of analysis should be guided by the following factors:

- frequency of incidents
- rate of disabling injuries
- severity potential
- new jobs

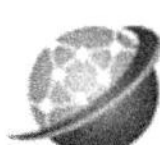

20) Answer A:

Many industry researchers have established and explored the notion of an "accident cycle" as the systemic series of events that ensures incidents continue to occur within a workplace, even though at many companies they may be few and far between. And because incidents tend to be sporadic and occur to individuals (rather than are frequent and occur to groups of people at once), leadership often fall into believing common misconceptions about the potential of better safety systems, and they often maintain their skepticism in spite of abundant counter-evidence. The accident cycle is characterized by a general series of events consequent of a *reactive* safety system and culture that is *top-down*—designed and enforced by leadership—rather than *bottom-up*—designed with input by frontline workers who hold themselves and each other accountable. R. Scott Stricoff describes the cycle succinctly: "When the recordable rate exceeds a facility's upper-limit perceived acceptability, management acts to drive the rate down. When the rate falls below that limit, attention to safety declines, and the recordable rate rises again. In this cycle, management action for improvement follows fluctuations in the injury frequency." when a safety system is *reactive* rather than *proactive*, the system *requires* incidents to occur to find where it needs improvement. And this therefore causes leadership as well as personnel to believe that a certain number of accidents may be allowable or acceptable—but thinking that the accidents occur only because the work is inherently dangerous, when in fact the safety system itself allows incidents to occur.

Domain 2 Quiz 3 Questions

1) According to current machine tools risk evaluation models, which of the following is true regarding the concept of "zero risk"?
   A) Zero risk is achievable given the correct task analysis was performed.
   B) Zero risk does not virtually exist.
   C) Zero risk can occur with the appropriate safety customs.
   D) Zero risk is the definitive goal of any safety program.

2) The risk remaining after preventive measures have been taken is called:
   A) Acceptable risk.
   B) Allowable risk.
   C) Unacceptable risk.
   D) Residual risk.

3) A study method that requires a multidisciplinary team, guided by an experienced leader and uses specific guide words (such as "no", "increase", "decrease", "reverse") that are systematically applied to parameters (e.g., temperature, pressure, flow) to identify the consequences of deviations (e.g., reduced flow) from design intent for various processes and operations is called a(n)?
   A) FTA.
   B) ETA.
   C) HAZOP.
   D) FMEA.

4) In a business or industrial setting, there are powerful reasons to focus on behavior before attitudes. These include all the following **except**
   A) A change in behavior can influence a change in attitude.
   B) A change in behavior does not influence a change in attitude.
   C) Behavior can be measured and therefore managed.
   D) Attitudes present measurement challenges.

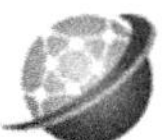

5) Basic principles of loss control include all the following **except:**
   A) "An unsafe act, an unsafe condition, and an accident are all symptomatic of something flawed in the management system."
   B) Certain sets of circumstances that will produce severe injuries can be predicted. These circumstances can be identified and controlled."
   C) "The key to effective line safety performance is management procedures that attach accountability."
   D) "Safety must be managed as a separate company function apart from the normal planning processes to assure management's commitment to safety and make it unmistakably evident to employees."

6) Reinforcement of desired behaviors is **best** accomplished by
   A) Cash incentives.
   B) Negative reinforcement at the work shift end.
   C) Positive reinforcement as soon as possible.
   D) It is not required as employees will change their behaviors only if they aspire to do so.

7) Which has the **greatest** impact or influences on behavior?
   A) Activators.
   B) Consequences.
   C) Discipline.
   D) Feedback.

8) Safety professionals demonstrate business acumen skills by incorporating the concept of cost effectiveness when advising management for risk based decision making. Which is a risk management principle applied when defining acceptable risk levels for machinery hazards?
   A) As low as reasonably achievable (ALARA).
   B) As low as reasonably practical (ALARP).
   C) Best Available Control Technology (BACT).
   D) Most Achievable Control Technology (MACT).

9) Safety professionals sometimes incorrectly use the terms risk and hazard interchangeably. Risk is **best** defined as:
   A) Conditions of things.
   B) Actions or inactions of people.
   C) A measure of the probability and severity of adverse effects.
   D) Any workplace condition that can result in injury, death, or property damage.

10) Which is a financial method for reducing the costs of accidents in an organization?
   A) Risk transfer.
   B) Risk projection.
   C) Financial risk management.
   D) Hierarchy of loss controls.

11) Failure Modes and Effects Analysis (FMEA) is a:
   A) Top down system safety technique.
   B) Bottom up system safety technique.
   C) Fault Tree system safety technique.
   D) Response management safety technique.

12) When presenting justifications for capital budget expenditures to decision makers, safety professionals frequently use cost-benefit analysis. A cost benefit analysis requires that:
   A) Project costs and benefits can be reasonably estimated in advance.
   B) Business units bearing the costs must be the same as those earning the benefits.
   C) Projects must be based on a minimal 10-year useful life.
   D) Financial professionals must approve and validate every assumption.

13) In behavior-based safety programs, Antecedent-Behavior-Consequence Analysis is often used to evaluate safety performance. In terms of consequences, the strongest and **most** powerful influences are:
   A) Soon, Uncertain, and Negative.
   B) Latent, Uncertain, and Positive.
   C) Soon, Certain, and Positive.
   D) Latent, Certain, and Negative.

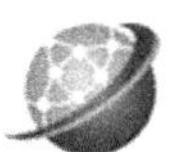

14) A company operates a fleet of estimators who work alone for most of the day traveling between several job sites. Can a behavior based safety (BBS) system be implemented for individual drivers?

A) Yes, by using a self-observation protocol.
B) Yes, by following each driver and recording their behaviors.
C) No, BBS is designed for peer to peer observation.
D) No, BBS only works for fixed locations with large groups of employees.

15) In order to select a system from among three potential safety design candidates, a Safety & Health consultant must recognize system failure will result in a loss, regardless of choice. An elementary design for each system showing probability of failure is shown below using standard "fault tree" symbols. Which system has the **lowest** overall failure probability?

A) System A has lower probability, and offers redundancy.
B) System B has lower probability, but has two potential single point failures.
C) System C is the simplest and has lowest probability.
D) The probability is the same for all three systems.

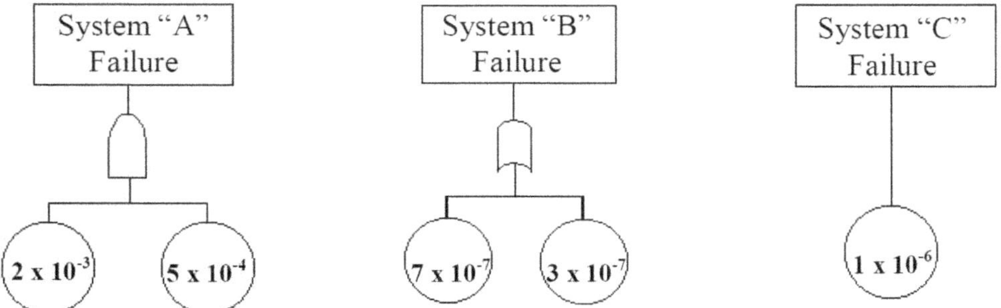

16) Risk can be expressed as the frequency of an event multiplied by the consequence of the event. Usually, consequence is expressed in units of monetary value used as a comparison of financial risk across different areas. Which of the following scenarios has the higher annual risk?

Scenario A: Minor employee injuries occur about twice per month and cost the company about $3,500 in lost work productivity and $2,500 in medical and insurance compensation per incident.

Scenario B: Catastrophic incidents occur about once every 30 years and cost the company about $1,200,000 in lost work productivity and equipment damage, along with $2,500,000 in legal fees and other compensation.

A) Scenario A has the higher risk.
B) Scenario B has the higher risk.
C) Scenarios A and B both have the same approximate risk.
D) Risk value for these scenarios show a frequency ratio of 1:2.

17) Which system has as its primary functions to identify hazardous conditions, assess their risk and establish effective risk control measures?

A) Risk control.
B) Risk management.
C) Loss control.
D) Loss management.

18) Which element is a risk management function?

A) Cause and effect analysis.
B) Supervisor first report of injury.
C) Identification and assessment.
D) Worker compensation experience modification rate.

19) A project is requiring long work hours for multiple weeks to meet a production deadline. You observe an equipment operator falling asleep between lifts, the **best** course of action is to:

A) Enter the operator on safety report.
B) Instruct the rigger to ensure the operator is awake.
C) Recommend to management to review work rest cycle.
D) Send an email or text reminding the operator of the importance of safety.

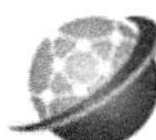

20) The **best** method to control a fall risk is:

A) Personal fall arrest system (PFAS) with harness and lanyard.
B) Safety net properly placed below the fall hazard area.
C) Guardrails to prevent access to the fall hazard.
D) Fall hazard warning signage.

Domain 2 Quiz 3 Answers

1) Answer B:

According to international standards on Machine tool safety such as ANSI B11 series and EN1050 (now ISO 14121), Zero Risk does not practically exist. The goal is to reduce risk to a tolerable level, then fully communicating any residual risk to the user. Hazards and their effects can best be identified by analyzing tasks and can be classified by the worst credible injury that may occur from a hazardous event.

The Risk is determined by estimating the severity of the hazard – and the probability of occurrence of a hazardous event

- Hazards and their effects can best be identified by analyzing tasks.
- Hazards can be classified by the worst credible injury that may occur from a hazardous event.
- Risk is determined by estimating the severity of the hazard – and the probability of occurrence of a hazardous event.

2) Answer D:

In ANSI Z10, risk is defined as an estimate of the combination of the likelihood of an occurrence of a hazardous event or exposure(s), and the severity of injury or illness that may be caused by the even or exposures. According to ANSI/ASSE/ISO Guide 73 (Z690.1-2011) Vocabulary for Risk Management, risk is simply the effect of uncertainty on objectives. Risk tolerance is an organizations readiness to bear the risk after risk treatment to achieve its objectives. Risk acceptance is an informed decision to take a risk. Acceptable risk is a residual risk level achieved after risk reduction measures have been applied. It is a risk level that is accepted for a given task (hazardous situation) or hazard. The terms "acceptable risk"; "retained risk" and "tolerable risk" are considered to be synonymous. Residual risk is defined as the risk remaining after preventive measures have been taken. No matter how effective the preventive actions, residual risk will always be present if a facility or operation continues to exist.

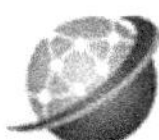

3) Answer C:

Hazard and operability study (HAZOP): Study used to identify problems associated with potential hazards and deviations in plant operations from the design specifications and is carried out by a multidisciplinary team following a structure that includes a series of guide words. When conducting a HAZOP, subject matter experts familiar with the process being studied are essential. A process hazard analysis leader familiar with the analytical method is important, but it is not essential for the study leader to be familiar with the process being studied. The purpose of a team leader is to challenge the logical thinking of the team.

4) Answer B:

According to "The Behavior Based Safety Process", a change in behavior does lead to a change in attitude.

5) Answer D:

According to Peterson's Techniques of Safety Management, only answers A, B, and C are representative of basic principles of loss control.

6) Answer C:

The two things needed for reinforcement of desired behaviors are to provide positive reinforcement and to keep reinforcement close in time to a specified behavior for a stronger effect. Some experts say to effect long term changes for minor infractions, a negative reinforcement may be utilized without overreacting. When discussing the "carrot and stick" management philosophy, some experts believe that the stick is no longer available, and the carrot is becoming less of an incentive.

7) Answer B:

All four answers have an impact on behavior, but consequences, in general, have the most impact. Discipline and feedback can be considered types of consequences, but there are others to be considered including positive reinforcement and reward. Activators are signals preceding behavior.

8) Answer B:
ALARP stands for As Low As Reasonably Practicable and promotes a management review, the intent of which is to achieve acceptable risk levels. Several depictions of the ALARP concept begin with an inverted triangle because it indicates that risk is greater at the top and much less at the bottom and is used in machinery risk assessments.
Use of the ALARA concept as a guideline originated in the atomic energy field and stands for as low as reasonably achievable and precedes the term ALARP. According to Nuclear Regulatory Commission, ALARA means making every reasonable effort to maintain exposures to ionizing radiation as far below the dose limits as practical.

9) Answer C:
A hazard is defined as a condition, set of circumstances, or inherent property that can cause injury, illness, or death. Risk is an estimation of the combination of the likelihood of an occurrence of a hazardous event or exposure(s), and the severity of injury or illness that may be caused by the event or exposures. Risk assessment is a process(s) used to evaluate the level of risk associated with hazards and system issues. A risk assessment matrix provides a qualitative method to categorize combinations of indicators for occurrence probability and severity outcome, thus establishing risk levels. A matrix provides an effective visual tool and helps in communication with decision makers when deciding on the actions to be taken to reduce the risk. Risk assessment matrices can also be used to compare and prioritize risks, and to effectively allocate mitigation resources. (ANSI/ASSE Z10-2012)

10) Answer A:
Several control techniques available are for treating loss exposures. The two categories for reducing the costs of accidents in an organization: prevention (loss control) and financial (cost reduction). Loss control techniques include engineering, administrative controls and personal protective equipment to deal with losses. Engineering controls include building a ventilation system to reduce explosive vapor levels, whereas administrative controls might limit exposures to toxic materials. Issuing personal protective equipment (PPE) such as respirators is the last line of defense against hazards in the workplace A company might try to avoid the loss altogether. Organizations can reduce exposure by substitution. Instead of mixing methylene chloride as a solvent ingredient in a commercial aerosol product a company could substitute a

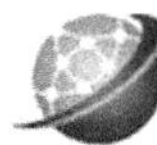

"safer" solvent to reduce the likelihood of a worker being exposed. ***Risk transfer*** assigns the liability to another party, rather than run the risk of loss itself. If methylene chloride mixing could not be accomplished safely in the plant, the company may choose to have the product shipped to a contractor who would mix the ingredient. If the contractor's workers are overcome by vapors from the solvent mixing, then the contractor would typically hold the liability. *Another form of risk transfer is insurance. Insurance* is designed to permit the company to shift the financial consequences of the risk to an insurance company. By paying the insurance company's *premiums*, the organization can expect specified *benefits* in the event of loss. With large numbers of insureds, insurance companies can more accurately estimate its own losses. Organizations may retain their loss exposures without dealing with them. This may be a result of ignorance or choice. Organizations that retain their own exposures may ignore them, or attempt to reduce them or they may, in fact, self-insure. Ignoring the risks may make the owners more confident, but dealing with the risks will make them more prepared for loss. Self-insurance is simply no insurance; the company retains the loss exposure. It should only be undertaken by companies with the financial resources necessary to absorb potential losses. (Friend & Kohn, 2007)

11) Answer B:

Failure mode and effects analysis (FMEA)—also "failure modes," plural, in many publications—was one of the first highly structured, systematic techniques for failure analysis. A FMEA is often the first step of a system reliability study. It involves reviewing as many components, assemblies, and subsystems as possible to identify failure modes, and their causes and effects. For each component, the failure modes and their resulting effects on the rest of the system are recorded in a specific FMEA worksheet. There are numerous variations of such worksheets. A FMEA can be a qualitative analysis, but may be put on a quantitative basis when mathematical failure rate models are combined with a statistical failure mode ratio database. Sometimes FMEA is extended to FMECA (Failure mode, effects, and criticality analysis) to indicate that criticality analysis is performed too. FMEA is an inductive reasoning (forward logic) single point of failure analysis and is a core task in reliability engineering, safety engineering and quality engineering. Quality engineering is especially concerned with the "Process" (Manufacturing and Assembly) type of FMEA. A successful FMEA activity helps to identify potential failure modes based on experience with similar products and processes—or based on common physics of failure logic. It is widely used in development and manufacturing industries in various phases of the product life cycle. Effects analysis refers to studying the consequences of those failures on different system levels. Functional analyses are needed as an input to determine correct failure modes, at all system levels, both for functional FMEA or Piece-Part (hardware) FMEA. An FMEA is used to structure Mitigation for Risk reduction based on either failure (mode) effect severity reduction or based on lowering the probability of failure or both. The FMEA is in principle a full inductive (forward logic) analysis, however the failure probability can only be estimated or reduced by understanding the failure mechanism. Ideally this probability shall be lowered to "impossible to occur" by eliminating the (root) causes. It is therefore important to include in the FMEA an appropriate depth of information on the causes of failure (deductive analysis)

12) Answer A:

Costs need to be expressed in terms that are useful. Expressing costs in the right terms can help people understand the importance of safety and its contribution to company profit. Although each level may have a preferred way of expressing cost data, it can help first-line supervisors and workers understand the importance of safety, and if expressions of cost are understood by workers, they are certainly understandable by managers. A popular way to justify business expenditures is by comparing the cost of some expenditure with the benefit achieved in financial terms. In cost-benefit analysis, the dollar values of all benefits and costs connected with program alternatives are estimated and then compared. Not all cost and benefits can be converted to quantitative terms; some may be expressed only qualitatively. A final decision applies both to quantitative and qualitative factors. (Brauer, 2006)

13) Answer C:

This is an essential tool of safety management for discovering and addressing the root causes of accidents. Applied behavior analysis helps the organization to assess the factors that are really driving its safety efforts.
ABC analysis involves the following principles:

- Both antecedents and consequences influence behavior,
- Consequences influence behavior powerfully and directly, and
- Antecedents (activators, triggers) influence behavior indirectly, primarily serving to predict consequences.

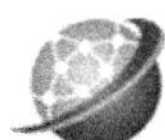

- The highest level of performance you can expect from the people you supervise is determined by the minimum standards you have established and maintained.
- Actions influence performance: Remember that silence (failure to act) is consent.

This non-punitive approach characterizes the discussions and interviews with workers, developing a list of triggers or antecedents of the at-risk behavior. ABC Analysis has three fundamental steps:

1. Analyze the At-risk Behavior
2. Analyze the Safe Behavior
3. Draft the Action Plan

When a facility's safety effort is not working it is the consequences in favor of safe behavior are weaker than the consequences in favor of at-risk behavior. There are three features that determine which consequences are stronger than others. The strongest behavioral consequences that are "soon, certain, and positive".

- **Timing.** A consequence that follows soon after a behavior influences behavior more effectively than consequences that occurs later. Again, silence is consent, thus failing to correct the unsafe act or at risk behavior gives employees the indication that their behavior is acceptable and the behavior goes uncorrected. This may set precedence for continued at risk behaviors. In an effective safety program, the at-risk behavior is identified and corrected immediately and effectively through immediate resolution of the antecedents.

- **Consistency.** A consequence that is certain to follow a behavior influences behavior more powerfully than an unpredictable or uncertain consequence. Failure to respond to each at risk behavior or failure to consistently reinforce the standard of performance will send mixed signals to employees. Prompt, consistent, and persistent corrective action is required. In any safety cultural change implementation, it is essential that all members of the team be informed of the consequence for at risk behavior, and that supervision enforces the rules. This lays the groundwork for predictable consequence.

- **Significance.** A positive consequence influences behavior more powerfully than a negative consequence. Punitive verses resolution: Resolution comes in the form of discussion, investigation of the behavior, in search of the underlying causes or antecedents that may have given the employee the misguided perception that has created the at-risk behavior. By talking with the employee and altering the perception, we have educated the employee without punitive action and have gained by-in for safe behavior.

Many safety programs are oriented toward penalties and punishments, rather like the traffic citation for speeding. The usual effect is not to change behavior, but rather to teach people not to get caught. Negative consequences are less powerful in their impact on worker behavior than positive consequences are. (Krause, 1997)

14) Answer A:

Behavior-based safety systems (BBS) typically use peer-to-peer observation methods to assess and measure conformance with behavior expectations. However, a self-observation protocol can be developed and implemented. It is important that the self-observed are involved in program design and development for successful implementation and buy in to how the data will be used. The primary goal for any safety program is to cultivate safer workers. Safer workers are a result of behavior change, in that workers recognize unsafe or at risk behaviors for what they are and then perform or do things to reduce or eliminate the at risk behavior.

15) Answer D:

System "A" is a parallel system, that is both the first **AND** the second components must fail to produce a system failure. To determine probability for a parallel system individual probabilities are multiplied.

$$(2 \times 10^{-3}) \times (5 \times 10^{-4}) = 1 \times 10^{-6}$$

System "B" is a series system, that is, if either the first **OR** the second components fail a system failure will occur. For components in series the total failure rate is the sum of individual components' failure rates.

$$(7 \times 10^{-7}) + (3 \times 10^{-7}) = 1 \times 10^{-6}$$

System "C" has only one component. Thus, the probability of system failure is the same as single component probability of failure.

$$1 \times 10^{-6}$$

Since the severity and probability for each system is the same, the loss risk is

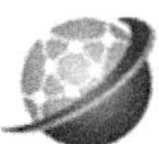

also the same. Given this situation, the selection process would consider overall system cost, deliverability, quality, longevity, human factors, etc.

16) Answer A:
These are essentially equivalent; however, Scenario A is a slightly higher risk.
Step One Calculate the cost of Minor incidents per year
The minor incidents cost the company $144,000 annually ($6,000 per incident multiplied by 24 times per year).
Step Two Calculate the cost of Major Incidents per year
The major incidents only happen once every 30 years, but cost $3,700,000 when they do occur. Dividing this over 30 years yields an annual risk exposure for the catastrophic incident of $123,333.

17) Answer C:
Loss control is the proactive measures taken to prevent or reduce **loss** evolving from accident, injury, illness and property damage. The aim of the **loss control** is to reduce the frequency and severity of losses. **Loss control** is directly related to human resource management, engineering and risk management practices.

18) Answer C:
Understanding the risk management function of an organization is important to the overall success of the safety management program.
Risk management is the process by which assessed risks are mitigated, minimized, or controlled through engineering, management, or operational means. This involves the optimal allocation of available resources in support of safety, performance, cost, and schedule.

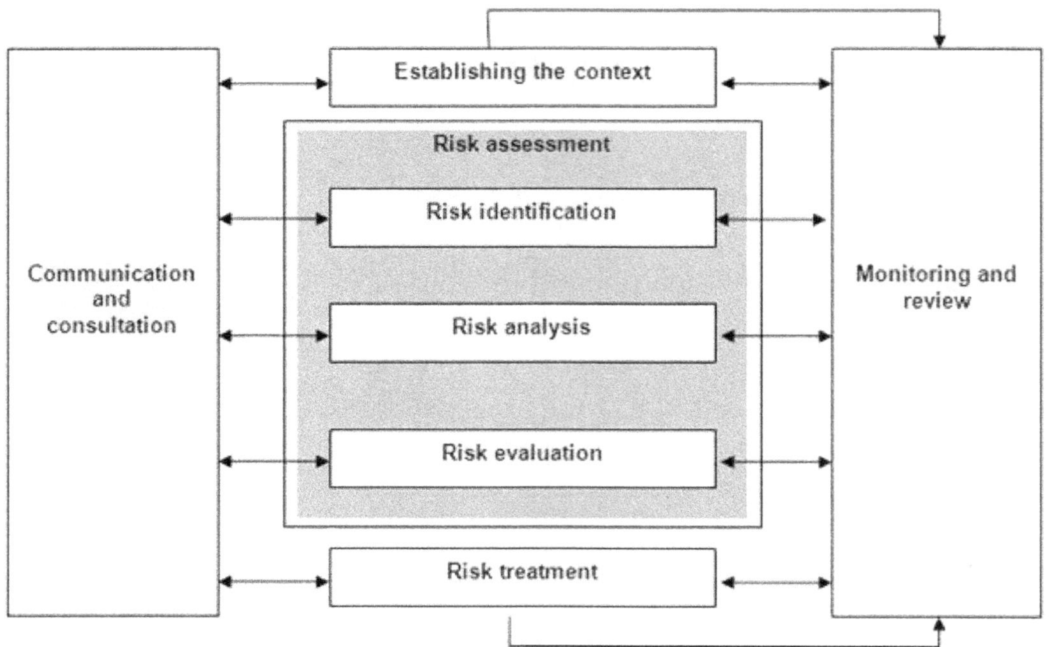

Risk assessment is the process of determining the risk presented by the identified hazards. This involves evaluating the identified hazard causal factors. Risk is defined as the combination of the severity of a defined exposure with its frequency of occurrence. The technique that effectively decreases a project's schedule risk without increasing the overall risk is to incorporate slack time into the project's critical path schedule early in project planning.
Hazard: Any real or potential condition that can cause injury, illness, or death to personnel; damage to or loss of a system, equipment, or property; or damage to the environment. A potentially unsafe condition resulting from failures, malfunctions, external events, errors, or a combination thereof. A condition, set of circumstances or inherent property that can cause injury, illness or death
Probability: The likelihood of a hazard causing an incident or exposure that could result in harm or damage for a selected unit of time, events, population, items or activities being considered.
Severity: The extent of harm or damage that could result from a hazard related incident or exposures.
Risk analysis is the process of identifying safety risk. This involves identifying hazards that present mishap risk with an assessment of the risk and then characterizing the risk as the product of the hazard severity times the hazard probability. Processes used to evaluate the level of risk associated with hazards and system issues.

- Assure Management commitment, involvement and direction (an Absolute)

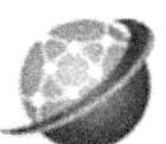

- Select a risk assessment team, including employees with knowledge of jobs and tasks.
- Establish the analysis parameters.
- Select a risk assessment technique.
- Identify the hazards.
- Consider failure modes.
- Assess the severity of consequences.
- Determine the occurrence probability, prominently taking into consideration the exposures.
- Define the initial risk
- Make risk acceptance or non-acceptant decisions with employee involvement.
- If needed, select and implement hazard avoidance, elimination, reduction and control measures.
- Address the residual risk.
- Document the results
- Follow-up on the actions taken

Root cause analysis (RCA) Process of identifying the basic lowest level causal factors for an event. Usually the event is an undesired event, such as a hazard or mishap.

Safety is freedom from those conditions that can cause death, injury, occupational illness, damage to or loss of equipment or property, or damage to the environment. The ability of a system to exclude certain undesired events (i.e., mishaps) during stated operation under stated conditions for a stated time. The ability of a system or product to operate with a known and accepted level of mishap risk. A built-in system characteristic.

Exposure: Contact with or proximity to a hazard, taking into account duration and intensity.

Risk communication is the interactive process of exchanging risk information and opinions among stakeholders.

Unacceptable risk: That risk that cannot be tolerated.

Acceptable risk: That part of identified mishap risk that is allowed to persist without taking further engineering or management action to eliminate or reduce the risk, based on knowledge and decision making. The system user is consciously exposed to this risk. A risk level achieved after risk reduction measures have been applied. It is a risk level that is accepted for a given task (hazardous situation) or hazard. The terms "acceptable risk" and "tolerable risk" are synonymous.

Accepted risk: Accepted risk has two parts: (1) risk that is knowingly understood and accepted by the system developer or user and (2) risk that in not known or understood and is accepted by default.
Residual risk: Overall risk remaining after system safety mitigation efforts have been fully implemented. It is, according to MIL-STD-882D, "the remaining mishap risk that exists after all mitigation techniques have been implemented or exhausted, in accordance with the system safety design order of precedence." Residual risk is the sum of all risk after mishap risk management has been applied. This is the total risk passed on to the user.
Mitigation is an action taken to reduce the risk presented by a hazard, by modifying the hazard to decrease the mishap probability and/or the mishap severity. Mitigation is generally accomplished through design measures, use of safety devices, warning devices, training, or procedures. It is also referred to as hazard mitigation and risk mitigation.
As low as reasonably practical (ALARP) Level of mishap risk that has been established and is considered as low as reasonably possible and still acceptable. It is based on a set of predefined ALARP conditions and is considered acceptable.
Mishap is an unplanned event or series of events resulting in death, injury, occupational illness, damage to or loss of equipment or property, or damage to the environment

19) Answer C:
The professional role of a risk/safety manager is to implement and evaluate the effectiveness of risk management program and report finding and recommendations to decision makers and key shareholders. Communication is a vital management component to any organization. Whether the purpose is to update employees on new policies, to prepare for a weather disaster, to ensure safety throughout the organization or to listen to the attitudes of employees, effective communication is an integral issue in effective management.

20) Answer C:
"Unprotected sides and edges." Each employee on a walking/working surface (horizontal and vertical surface) with an unprotected side or edge which is 6 feet (1.8 m) or more above a lower level shall be protected from falling by the use of guardrail systems, safety net systems, or personal fall arrest systems. Barriers or guardrail systems are a preventative engineering control as compared to an administrative or PPE control.

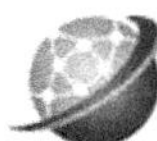

Domain 3: Safety, Health, and Environmental Concepts

Domain 3: Safety, Health, and Environmental Concepts 33.1%
Knowledge of: 1. Concepts in the Globally Harmonized System of Classification and Labeling of Chemicals (GHS) 2. Common controls for slips, trips, and falls (from all levels) 3. Common controls for working with electricity 4. Common controls for working in confined spaces 5. Common controls for working around machinery and equipment 6. Common controls for bloodborne pathogens 7. Common controls for lead 8. Common controls for asbestos 9. Common controls for radiation (ionizing and non-ionizing) 10. Common controls for temperature extremes (e.g., cold or heat stress, contact with extreme temperatures, thermal stress) 11. Common controls for vibration (e.g., whole body, hand/arm) 12. Common controls for noise 13. Common controls for ergonomic hazards associated with the type of work, body positions, or strain on the body from working conditions (e.g., improperly adjusted workstations/chairs, frequent lifting, awkward movements, poor posture, repetitive movements, use of too much force, compression) 14. Common controls for any form of chemical hazards (e.g., liquids, vapors, fumes, dusts, gases, flammable liquids, and pesticides) 15. Common controls for workplace stressors (e.g., workload demand, fatigue, harassment, lack of schedule flexibility, lack of control) 16. Occupational health programs (e.g., medical surveillance, fit for duty, return to work, substance abuse testing)

Skill to:

1. Recognize unsafe conditions or acts that can cause slips, trips, and falls (from all levels)
2. Recognize unsafe conditions or acts when working with electricity
3. Recognize unsafe conditions or acts when working in confined spaces
4. Recognize unsafe conditions or acts when working around machinery and equipment (e.g., caught in, struck by, pinch points)
5. Recognize conditions that could lead to unsafe exposures to molds and allergens
6. Recognize unsafe conditions or acts related to potential exposures to bloodborne pathogens
7. Recognize unsafe conditions or acts related to potential exposures lead
8. Recognize unsafe conditions or acts related to potential exposures to asbestos
9. Recognize unsafe conditions or acts related to potential exposures to radiation (ionizing and non-ionizing)
10. Recognize unsafe conditions or acts related to potential exposures to temperature extremes (e.g., cold or heat stress, contact with extreme temperatures, thermal stress)
11. Recognize unsafe conditions or acts related to potential exposures to vibration (e.g., whole body, hand/arm)
12. Recognize unsafe conditions or acts related to potential exposures to noise
13. Recognize unsafe conditions or acts related to ergonomic hazards associated with the type of work, body positions, or strain on the body from working conditions (e.g., improperly adjusted workstations/chairs, frequent lifting, awkward movements, poor posture, repetitive movements, use of too much force, compression)
14. Recognize unsafe conditions or acts related to exposures to any form of chemicals (e.g., liquids, vapors, fumes, dusts, gases, flammable liquids, and pesticides)
15. Recognize unsafe conditions or acts related to workplace stressors (e.g., workload demand, fatigue, harassment, lack of schedule flexibility, lack of control)

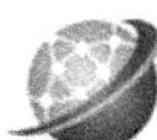

Hazard Prevention and Control

Effective prevention and control of workplace hazards is critical to protecting employee safety and health and avoiding workplace incidents. Prevention and control allows employers to minimize or eliminate safety and health risks and liabilities as well as meet their legal obligation to provide employees with a safe and healthy work environment. Hazard prevention and control reduces costs, improves efficiency, and boosts product or service quality. They can also help improve an organization's relationships with its stakeholders and enhance its image as a responsible organization.

Hazards can only be prevented or controlled after they have been identified. Therefore, most hazard prevention and control takes place after workplace hazards have been systematically identified and assessed. If the hazard identification process finds serious hazards that are not yet controlled, employers should implement interim controls without delay and investigate further options during the hazard prevention and control process.
Hazard prevention and control is an ongoing process. Prevention and control measures are periodically assessed, and changes or updates are made as needed to ensure that these measures continue to be effective in light of changing control technologies or changing workplace conditions.

Effective control techniques are often easy to identify and implement for common and well understood workplace hazards. However, many hazards and control options need to be examined in more detail. For example, the best control options for more serious and complicated hazards may not be self-evident. In such cases, employers often use interim controls until they have identified, implemented, and selected more permanent control options. Where possible, selected hazard control methods should address root causes and be effective both upon implementation and in the long term.

Hazard prevention and control consists of:

- Identify control options and select controls.
- Select controls to protect employees during emergencies.
- Implement controls according to the priorities established during hazard identification and assessment.
- Track progress, verify implementation, and evaluate effectiveness.

Identify Control Options and Select Controls

Hazard prevention and control begins with gathering information to understand how *all* identified workplace hazards can be prevented and controlled. For many hazards, several control options are usually available and it is valuable to examine the pros and cons of each. Prevention and control information can be obtained from many sources, including regulatory and consensus standards and technical guidance, industry trade and professional associations, safety-related publications, and equipment and service vendors and suppliers. Employees often provide valuable input. They may have seen or heard of control measures being used elsewhere, and they may be able to suggest unique solutions based on their familiarity with the facility, equipment, and work processes.

Once decision makers understand what options are available, they evaluate and select the most effective and feasible measures for their workplace. This involves considering questions such as:

- What safety and health risks exist in the workplace?
- Where and how do these risks occur?
- What types of emergencies could arise, and what safety and health risks would they pose?
- What are appropriate risk reduction goals?
- What risk control technologies are available?
- How cost effective are these technologies?
- What do federal and state standards require?
- What internal standards does our organization have?
- What are current best practices within our industry?

Where appropriate, employers sometimes consult with qualified safety and health professionals (such as Certified Industrial Hygienists or Certified Safety Professionals) to gain additional information and perspective as they consider these types of questions and examine options. Engineering controls are the most effective because they reduce reliance on human factors to achieve protection. Other types of controls should be considered in the order listed to provide additional protection when engineering controls alone are insufficient.

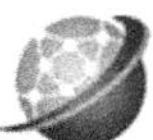

Hierarchy of Controls[22]

In applying a hierarchy of controls, the desired outcome of actions taken is to achieve an acceptable risk level. Acceptable risk is that risk for which the probability of a hazards-related incident or exposure occurring and the severity of harm or damage that could result are as low as reasonably practicable (ALARP) and tolerable in the situation being considered. That definition requires several factors be taken into consideration:

- avoiding, eliminating or reducing the probability of a hazards-related incident or exposure occurring
- reducing the severity of harm or damage that may result if an incident or exposure occurs
- the feasibility and effectiveness of risk-reduction measures to be taken, and their costs, in relation to the amount of risk reduction to be achieved

Decision makers should understand that with respect to the six levels of action shown in the following hierarchy of controls the methods described in the first, second and third action levels are more effective because they:

- are preventive actions that eliminate/reduce risk by design, substitution and engineering measures;
- rely the least on the performance of personnel;
- are less defeat able by supervisors or workers

Actions described in the fourth, fifth and sixth levels are contingent actions and rely greatly on the performance of personnel for their effectiveness. The following hierarchy of controls is considered state-of-the-art, and it is compatible with the hierarchy in ANSI/ASSE Z10-2012:

1. Eliminate or reduce risks in the design and redesign processes.
2. Reduce risks by substituting less hazardous methods or materials.
3. Incorporate engineering controls.
4. Provide warning systems
5. Apply administrative controls
6. Provide PPE.

The hierarchy provides a systematic way to determine the most effective feasible method to reduce risk associated with a hazard. When controlling the hazard, first consider methods to eliminate the hazard. This is best accomplished in the concept and design phase of a project.

[22] Adapted from ANSI Z10-2012 Occupational Safety and Health Management Systems.

Implement Controls According to the Priorities

Once hazard prevention and control measures have been selected, they need to be implemented. The first step is to develop a written implementation plan. Implementation plans typically specify, for example:

- What hazards need control?
- What measures will be implemented?
- In what order?
- Who will implement them?
- By when?
- Should a written operating procedure (for example, standard operating procedure (SOPs), or JSA/JHAs) be developed?
- What employee training is needed?
- When and how will implementation be confirmed?
- When and how will effectiveness be evaluated?
- When and how will routine inspections be conducted to ensure that hazard prevention and control measures remain operational?
- When and how will preventive maintenance be conducted?

In more advanced OHSMSs, a written plan helps ensure that managers and employees have a roadmap for effective implementation. It also provides a framework that management can use to track progress.

When resources are limited, employers may not be able to implement all desired controls at once. In these cases, employers should, where feasible, implement measures on a "worst-first" basis according to the hazard ranking priorities established during hazard identification and risk assessment. In other words, measures that protect employees from the highest priority hazards are implemented first, followed by controls for other hazards, in order of decreasing priority. Interim controls are implemented as necessary to protect employees while permanent controls are not in place. Employers are also encouraged to rapidly implement all measures that are easy and inexpensive, regardless of the level of hazard they control.

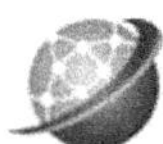

In an effective OHSMS, implementation will be tracked and verified. For example:

- Have all control measures been implemented according to schedule?
- Have engineering controls been properly installed and tested?
- Have employees been appropriately trained?
- Do all employees understand the controls, including safe work practices and PPE use requirements?
- Are these controls being used correctly and consistently?

Regular inspections and routine preventive maintenance will be needed on an ongoing basis to ensure that the control measures remain effective in preventing hazards. Regular inspections are important to confirm that (1) engineering controls are operating as designed and have not been removed or deactivated, and (2) work practices, administrative controls, and PPE use policies are being observed. Routine preventive maintenance of equipment, facilities, and controls helps provide ongoing prevention of incidents due to equipment failure. For example, maintaining the moving parts of machinery ensures that a part does not fail and turn into a flying object that can injure an employee.

Organizations that want to achieve a more robust OHSMS do more original research and study of available control options. Some control measures may be crafted based on detailed engineering studies or employee exposure monitoring and occupational health screening. Employers often consult with qualified internal and external professionals. Organizations begin to play a leadership role within professional and trade associations and are comfortable sharing information on control measures. Operational control plans are developed for all identified hazards, with detailed instructions and implementation and inspection plans. Training in control measures is more formal and frequent, and training effectiveness is evaluated. The organization's emergency response plan is more detailed and expansive. Drills and tests are conducted more frequently and are coordinated with external emergency responders.

Domain 3 Quiz 1 Questions

1) The **primary** benefit of using a data logger in conjunction with industrial hygiene monitoring devices is that it
   A) Manually records data.
   B) Codes the data so it can't be read without the code.
   C) Digitize data for future use and analysis.
   D) Industrial hygiene does not need to be monitored.

2) Hazardous waste profiles from a several chemical processes yield non-potable water, lithium metal, acetone and halogenated hydrocarbons. What is the **greatest** concern for a waste site worker segregating waste streams into 55 gal drums?
   A) Mixing lithium metal and non-potable water.
   B) Mixing lithium metal and acetone.
   C) Mixing spent acetone and non-potable water.
   D) Mixing halogenated hydrocarbons and acetone.

3) In product development, manufacture and use, which phase is **most** important to guarantee a safe product is provided to the consumer?
   A) Design.
   B) Testing.
   C) Production.
   D) Maintenance.

4) When conducting a preliminary hazard evaluation for a new process, which question is **least appropriate** during this phase of analysis?
   A) What are the raw materials?
   B) What intermediate products are formed in the process?
   C) What by-products may be released?
   D) When should you provide PPE?

5) If a small mobile crane with rubber tires has struck a power line and is apparently dead, lying across the crane boom, what is the **best** course of action for the crane operator?
   A) Jump from crane and run away.
   B) Stay in crane until the emergency crew arrives.
   C) Have oiler knock power line from the boom with a wood pole.
   D) Swing boom back and forth until line breaks or falls off.

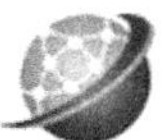

6) Approach to infection control to treat all human blood and certain human body fluids as if they were known to be infectious for HIV, HBV and other bloodborne pathogens is called:
   A) Exposure control plan.
   B) Contamination prevention.
   C) Exposure Incident.
   D) Universal Precautions.

7) The three distinct parts of a "means of egress" include
   A) Exit access, exit, and exit discharge.
   B) Door, passageway, and ramps.
   C) Door opening device, door, and exit light.
   D) Horizontal exits, stairs, and ramps.

8) An electrical conduit that is very warm to the touch is discovered during an industrial safety inspection. Which of the following descriptions **best** fits this condition?
   A) Conduit is hot with electric energy due to a ground fault.
   B) Conduits are always warm to the touch.
   C) Conduit is likely absorbing radiant heat from the furnace.
   D) Conduit likely contains overloaded electrical wiring.

9) Safety Data Sheets (SDS) for chemicals in the work area shall be readily accessible during to workers in a reasonable amount of time. The **most effective** way to maintain updated SDSs for the entire facility is to:
   A) Distribute all facility SDSs to each worker by email and place printed copies in each work area.
   B) Maintain a master printed copy of all SDSs in the safety office and make available on request.
   C) Provide an external hard drive in each work area with copies of all the facility SDSs.
   D) Integrate an automated electronic SDS updates from suppliers with cloud-based searchable databases synced with worker smart phones.

10) A facility is installing a new machine as part of their operations. The new equipment consists of two rollers rotating inward, creating a pinch point. The **best** option for protecting operators from this hazard is:
   A) Installation of a fixed guard with interlocks.
   B) Proper training to safely bypass a removable guard.
   C) Use of distance to prevent worker exposure.
   D) Install pull-back hand restraints.

11) Insulated enclosures are often used in noise control and designed **primarily** to:
   A) Eliminate the source from generating sound pressure levels.
   B) Reduce noise level at the point of sound wave generation.
   C) Reduce noise exposure with sound pressure level absorbing materials.
   D) Amplify sound pressure levels between source and the barrier.

12) A ____________________consists of all equipment used to keep an employee from reaching a fall point, such as the edge of an elevated working surface.
   A) Fall restraint system.
   B) Fall protection system.
   C) Fall arrest system.
   D) Safety net system.

13) Which of the following are the GHS signal words that indicate the relative degree of a hazard's severity?
   A) Danger, Warning.
   B) Caution, Danger.
   C) Hazardous, Dangerous.
   D) Warning, Caution.

14) Effective hazard communication programs for workers using chemicals require:
   A) GHS training, labels, chemical hazard analysis, and Safety Data Sheets.
   B) Safety Data Sheets, chemical inventories, audits, and training.
   C) Bi lingual labels, chemical hazard analysis, chemical inventories, and GHS training.
   D) Hazard classifications, Safety Data Sheets, labels, and training.

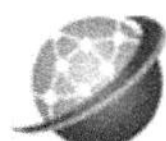

15) All Safety Data Sheets are comprised of
  A) 10 sections.
  B) 12 sections.
  C) 14 sections.
  D) 16 sections.

16) The pictogram represents which hazard?
  A) Pyrophorics and explosives.
  B) Narcotic effects.
  C) Reproductive toxicity.
  D) Acute toxicity and narcotic effects.

17) The **first** action to be considered in the hierarchy of control is:
  A) Training of workers based on job hazard analysis.
  B) Prevention by risk avoidance through hazard elimination.
  C) Issue personal protective equipment for risk reduction.
  D) Hazardous substitution through risk transfer.

18) The machine presents a serious hazard if the belt is not guarded. There are four situations that could contribute to an accident or injury. Which Boolean expression could result in an injury to the machinist?
  A=The belt guard is not in position.
  B=The belt severs.
  C=The belt is compromised by an external source.
  D=The belt guard will protect the machinist.

  A) BD+CD
  B) AB+AC
  C) CD+BD
  D) (A+B)D+BC

19) Professionals devoted to the art and science of anticipation, recognition, evaluation and control of those environmental factors in the workplace that may cause impaired health are:
  A) Industrial Hygienists.
  B) Industrial Toxicologists.
  C) Health Physicists.
  D) Medical Pathologists.

20) Which of the following are techniques for controlling worker radiation exposure?
   A) Exposure Time, PPE, and shielding.
   B) Exposure type, ionizing and non-ionizing.
   C) Exposure Time, distance from source, and shielding.
   D) Low Exposure, achievable practices, and source reduction.

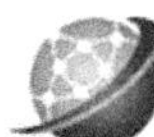

Domain 3 Quiz 1 Answers

1) Answer C:

A data logger is an electronic instrument used to take measurements from sensors and store those measurements for future use. Some common measurements include temperature, pressure, current, velocity, strain, displacement and other physical phenomena.
A data logger works with sensors to convert physical phenomena and stimuli into electronic signals such as voltage or current. These electronic signals are then converted or digitized into binary data. The binary data is then easily analyzed by software and stored on a PC hard drive or on other storage media such as memory cards. The ability to take sensor measurements and store the data for future use is, by definition, a characteristic of a data logger. However, a data-logging application rarely requires only data acquisition and storage. Inevitably, you need the ability to analyze and present the data to determine results and make decisions based on the logged data.

2) Answer A:

The consequences of mixing incompatible chemicals together are potentially severe from a health and safety perspective. From a disposal perspective, mixing of wastes can be costly. Mixed wastes can result in the need for sequential treatment using different technologies at different facilities. It is unlikely that random mixing of different waste materials together will reduce the toxicity of the mixture. Lithium metal is water reactive and should not be mixed.

3) Answer A:

According to Willie Hammer in "*Product Safety Management and Engineering*", management responsibilities throughout the process is the most important, however during the design phase, the designers are the most important in producing a safe product.

4) Answer D:

According to the "Fundamentals of Industrial Hygiene" the initial hazard recognition process, includes the following are questions; what are the raw materials? what is produced?; what intermediate products are formed in the process?; what by-products may be released?; what are the usual cleaning or maintenance procedures at the end of the day, end of a run or changeover to another product?; and what hazardous waste is produced and how is it disposed of?

5) Answer B:

Each power line contact situation poses different problems. However, the generally accepted guidance is for the crane operator to stay in the cab until power company emergency crews arrive. Often power lines are equipped with fault clearing re-closers, which will reapply power to a faulted line after a few minutes. The re-closer can cycle three or four times before the line is really disconnected and then it is still unsafe because of cross feed situations. Departing the cab should only be considered if a fire or other situation requires it. Jumping from the cab with feet together is the only safe departure method. Contact must be avoided with the energized crane and earth and step potential must be kept at a minimum.

6) Answer D:

OSHA 1910.1030(b) Bloodborne Pathogen Standard defines ***Exposure Incident*** as a specific eye, mouth, other mucous membrane, non-intact skin, or parenteral contact with blood or other potentially infectious materials that results from the performance of an employee's duties. **Universal precautions** are an approach to infection control to treat all human blood and certain human body fluids as if they were known to be infectious for HIV, HBV and other bloodborne pathogens. If exposures to blood or other body fluids are reasonably anticipated, you are required by the Occupational Safety and Health Administration (OSHA) Bloodborne Pathogens Standard to develop an **Exposure Control Plan.**

7) Answer A:

NFPA 101, Life Safety Code, states, "A means of egress is a continuous and unobstructed way of exit travel from any point in a building or structure to a public way and consists of three separate and distinct parts: (a) the exit access, (b) the exit, and (c) the exit discharge. A means of egress comprises the vertical and horizontal travel and shall include intervening room spaces, doorways, hallways, corridors, passageways, balconies, ramps, stairs, enclosures, lobbies, escalators, horizontal exits, courts, and yards.

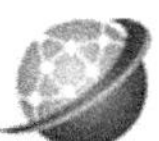

8) Answer D:

One of the most common causes of electrically created fires is overheated wiring because of overloading. Many factors contribute to a safe installation. The wire must be sized (correct gauge) properly to handle the current. Overcurrent protection (fuses or circuit breakers) must also be correctly sized and function properly. Additionally, electrical raceways must not be overloaded with electrical wiring. The sizing of wiring and the amount of wiring allowed for a given size of raceway is strictly regulated in the National Electrical Code. Generally, conduit will not feel hot to the touch even under severe circuit loading if installed according to code.

9) Answer D:

The most effective way is to post all Material Safety Data Sheets is by use of the company local area network (LAN) and a data base program. This allows updates to be posted when they are received and are available to all work areas as soon as they are posted.

10) Answer A:

If the pinch point in question does not require frequent access for maintenance or cleaning, the best answer is a permanent guard that makes removal difficult. Authors would choose a fixed guard.

11) Answer C:

According to the NSC Fundamentals of industrial Hygiene, generally, an enclosure is placed around a noise source to prevent noise from getting outside. Enclosures are normally lined with sound-absorption material to decrease internal sound pressure buildup. Another option is to enclose the worker, such as sound proof booths that prevent noise from getting inside.

12) Answer A:

The best selection is A because the definition of a fall restraint system consists of the equipment used to keep an employee from *reaching a fall point,* such as the edge of a roof or the edge of an elevated working surface. The most commonly utilized fall restraint system is a standard guardrail. A tie off system that "restrains" the employee from falling off an elevated working surface is another type of fall restraint.

Fall protection systems consist of:

- Guardrail Systems
- Safety Net Systems
- Personal Fall Arrest Systems
- Fall restraint system
- Positioning Device Systems
- Warning Line Systems
- Controlled Access Zones
- Safety Monitoring Systems
- Covers
- Protection From Falling Objects
- Fall Protection Plan (limited)

Personal Fall Arrest Systems must include 4 elements referred to as ABCD's of Fall Arrest:

- A - Anchorage - a fixed structure or structural adaptation, often including an anchorage connector, to which other components of PFAS are rigged.
- B - Body Wear - a full body harness worn by worker.
- C - Connector - a subsystem component connecting harness to anchorage - such as a lanyard.
- D - Deceleration Device - a subsystem component designed to dissipate forces associated with a fall arrest event.

13) Answer A:

The signal word indicates the relative degree of severity a hazard. The signal words used in GHS are

- "Danger" for more severe hazards.
- "Warning" for less severe hazards.

Signal words are standardized and assigned to hazard categories within endpoints. Some lower level hazard categories do not use signal words. Only one signal word corresponding to the class of the most severe hazard should be used on a label. The GHS hazard pictograms, signal word and hazard statements should be located together on the label. The actual label format or layout is not specified in GHS. National authorities may choose to specify where information should appear on the label or allow supplier discretion.

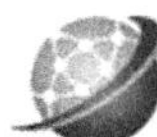

14) Answer D:
The OSHA Hazard Communication Standard (HCS) is now aligned with the Globally Harmonized System of Classification and Labeling of Chemicals (GHS). **In order to ensure chemical safety in the workplace, information about the identities and hazards of the chemicals must be available and understandable to workers. OSHA's Hazard Communication Standard (HCS) requires the development and dissemination of such information:**

- Chemical manufacturers and importers are required to evaluate the hazards of the chemicals they produce or import, and prepare labels and safety data sheets to convey the hazard information to their downstream customers;
- All employers with hazardous chemicals in their workplaces must have labels and safety data sheets for their exposed workers, and train them to handle the chemicals appropriately.

An effective Hazard Communication program shall include:
Hazard classification: Provides specific criteria for classification of health and physical hazards, as well as classification of mixtures.
Labels: Chemical manufacturers and importers are required to provide a label that includes a harmonized signal word, pictogram, and hazard statement for each hazard class and category. Precautionary statements must also be provided.
Safety Data Sheets: Specified 16-section format.
Information and training: Employers are required to train workers on the chemical labels elements and safety data sheets.

15) Answer D:
The SDS will include at least the following section numbers and headings and associated information within each heading, in the order listed:

- **Section 1 Identification**—includes product identifier, manufacturer or distributor name, address, phone number, emergency phone number, recommended use, and restrictions on use
- **Section 2 Hazard(s) identification**—includes all hazards regarding the chemical and required label elements
- **Section 3 Composition/Information on ingredients**—includes information on chemical ingredients and trade secret claims
- **Section 4 First-aid measures**—includes important acute or delayed symptoms or effects and required treatment
- **Section 5 Fire-fighting measures**—lists suitable extinguishing techniques, equipment, and chemical hazards from fire
- **Section 6 Accidental release measures**—lists emergency procedures, protective equipment, and proper methods of containment and cleanup
- **Section 7 Handling and storage**—lists precautions for safe handling and storage, including incompatibilities
- **Section 8 Exposure controls/Personal protection**—lists OSHA's permissible exposure limits, threshold limit values (TLVs), appropriate engineering controls, and personal protective equipment (PPE)
- Section 9 Physical and chemical properties—lists the chemical's characteristics
- **Section 10 Stability and reactivity**—lists chemical stability and possibility of hazardous reactions
- **Section 11 Toxicological information**—includes routes of exposure, related symptoms, acute and chronic effects, and numerical measures of toxicity
- Section 12 Ecological information*
- Section 13 Disposal considerations*
- Section 14 Transportation information*
- Section 15 Regulatory information*
- **Section 16 Other information**—includes date of preparation or last revision

*Notation concerning Sections 12 to 15: OSHA will not enforce information requirements in Sections 12 to 15; however, the SDS must include at least the heading names for those sections.

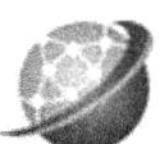

16) Answer D:

It is used on a chemical label for substances that represent the following hazards:

- Irritant–irritates the skin or eyes
- Skin sensitizer– an allergic response following skin contact
- Acute toxicity– a single short-term exposure may be fatal or cause organ damage
- Narcotic effects such as drowsiness, lack of coordination, and dizziness
- Respiratory tract irritation

The GHS symbols have been incorporated into pictograms for use on the GHS label. Pictograms include the harmonized hazard symbols plus other graphic elements, such as borders, background patterns or colors which are intended to convey specific information. The GHS hazard pictograms, signal word and hazard statements should be located together on the label.

GHS Pictograms and Hazard Classes		
▪ Oxidizers	▪ Flammables ▪ Self-Reactive ▪ Pyrophorics ▪ Self-Heating ▪ Emits Flammable Gas ▪ Organic Peroxides	▪ Explosives ▪ Self-Reactive ▪ Organic Peroxides
▪ Acute toxicity (severe)	▪ Corrosives	▪ Gases Under Pressure
▪ Carcinogen ▪ Respiratory Sensitizer ▪ Reproductive Toxicity ▪ Target Organ Toxicity ▪ Mutagenicity ▪ Aspiration Toxicity	▪ Environmental Toxicity	▪ Irritant ▪ Dermal Sensitizer ▪ Acute toxicity (harmful) ▪ Narcotic Effects ▪ Respiratory Tract ▪ Irritation

17) Answer B:

Risks are reduced to an acceptable level through the application of the hierarchy of controls. A hierarchy of controls provides a systematic way of thinking, considering steps in a ranked and sequential order, to choose the most effective means of eliminating or reducing hazards and their associated risks. Acknowledging that premise that risk reduction measures should be considered and taken in a prescribed order represents an important step in the evolution of the practice of safety. These methods are to be applied when new facilities, equipment and processes are acquired; when existing facilities, equipment and processes are altered; and when incidents are investigated.

18) Answer B:

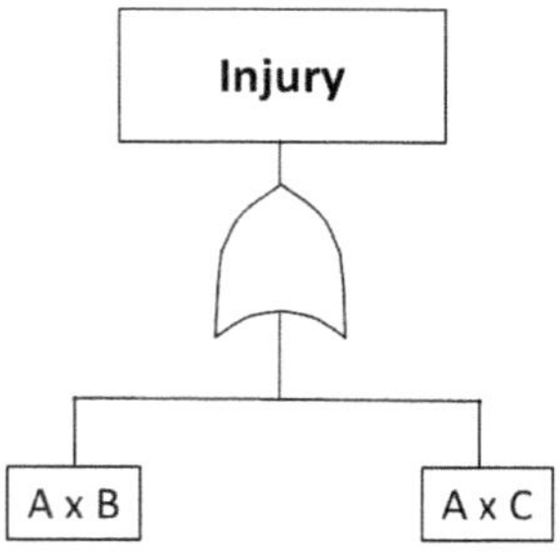

This may be easier to see in a small fault tree. Determine the condition that could result in an injury, in this case A and B or A and C have to exist and either situation will produce an injury, therefore an OR gate.

19) Answer A:

According to the Fundamental of Industrial Hygiene, an **Industrial Toxicologist** is one who studies the harmful, or toxic, properties of substances and determines dose thresholds. An **Industrial Hygienist** is one devoted to the art and science of anticipation, recognition, evaluation and control of those environmental factors in the workplace that may cause sickness, impaired health and well-being. A **Health Physicist** studies the field of science concerned with radiation physics and radiation biology with the goal of providing technical information and proper techniques regarding safe use of ionizing radiation. **Pathologists** are physicians who diagnose and characterize disease in living patients by examining biopsies or bodily fluid. Pathologists may also conduct autopsies to investigate causes of death.

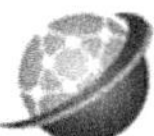

20) Answer C:

Radiation is energy that comes from a source and travels through space at the speed of light. This energy has an electric field and a magnetic field associated with it, and has wave-like properties. Protection from radiation involves time, distance, and shielding. Controlling worker exposure by minimizing the time of exposure to as low as reasonably achievable (ALARA) and/or increasing the distance from the radioactive source and/or using shielding.

Shielding is a barrier that protects workers from harmful radiations released by radioactive materials. Lead bricks, dense concrete, water, and earth are examples of materials used for shielding. Radiation containment is an important component for controlling radiation exposure. Containment of radiation contamination should be monitored and detected. To control radiation

TYPE	EFFECTS	SHIELDING
Alpha	Short range -- <4" in air Chemically similar to calcium (can collect in kidneys, bones, liver, lungs & spleen) Eyes are an internal exposure	Skin, paper, thin film of water
Beta	Secondary release of gamma radiation Higher energies can cause skin burns	Light metals (like aluminum)
Neutron	Secondary release of gamma radiation	Carbon or high Hydrogen content (like water)
Gamma & X-ray	Most penetrating Electromagnetic radiation – Gamma (natural) & X-ray (manmade)	Heavy metals (like lead)

Domain 3 Quiz 2 Questions

1) The incorporation of hazard analysis and risk assessment methods early in design and redesign processes and taking appropriate actions so risks of injury or damage are at an acceptable level is termed:
   A) Severity.
   B) Deterrence through design.
   C) Safety through design.
   D) Hierarchy of controls.

2) A Confined space is large enough and so configured that an employee can bodily enter and perform assigned work; not designed for continuous employee occupancy; and
   A) Has an hazardous atmosphere that impairs self-rescue.
   B) Has only one way in and one way out.
   C) Has limited or restricted means for entry or exit.
   D) Has an internal configuration that creates a trap.

3) In a confined space operation, it is required to control hazardous chemicals in a section of piping system, how **best** to control this hazard?
   A) Blanking and blinding.
   B) Inerting the space.
   C) Confined space permit.
   D) Double block and bleed.

4) The **proper** order of atmospheric testing in a confined space is:
   A) Flammability, oxygen, toxic.
   B) Toxic, oxygen, flammability.
   C) Oxygen, flammability, toxicity.
   D) Oxygen, toxics, flammability.

5) IR-B includes light wavelengths from 1.4 to 100μm. Infrared radiation can cause eye injury and **most likely** associated with which work environment?
   A) Dark room for photography.
   B) Microscope use in a laboratory.
   C) Foundry operations.
   D) X-ray technician.

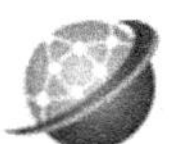

6) The signal word *"DANGER,"* on product warning labels is used where there is an immediate hazard and exposure that, if encountered, may result in:
   A) Death or severe personal injury.
   B) Death, severe personal injury, or extensive property damage.
   C) Death, extensive property damage, extensive product damage and severe personal injury.
   D) Death, loss of livelihood, and property damage.

7) The **primary** function of a warning sign is:
   A) To provide information for supervisors.
   B) To provide information for employees.
   C) For employees to recognize and understand hazards.
   D) To protect a company from regulatory citations and lawsuits.

8) Proof testing is defined as:
   A) A test that stretches the sling to its maximum tensile strength.
   B) A logic tree designed to help in selection of a proper sling.
   C) A chemical test to make certain the correct material was used to construct a sling.
   D) A nondestructive tension test performed by the sling manufacture or an equivalent entity to verify construction and workmanship of a sling.

9) New construction work is being conducted on an interior room on a high floor of a building. The top, floor, east and west walls are constructed. The North South walls are tarped off with a kerosene heating unit is in the space what is the **most** appropriate action?
   A) Rotate work crew in and out.
   B) Monitor the atmosphere.
   C) Remove the heating fuel.
   D) Supply Fresh air flow.

10) A company is setting up a laboratory to do experimental work for their electroplating division. One workstation involves use of perchloric acid. Management plans on purchasing a local exhaust hood for this station and reviewing recommendations on hood specifications. Which recommendation is of the **greatest** concern?

A) Hood and duct material must be non-reactive, acid resistant and relatively impervious.
B) Hood and duct should be designed for easy cleaning and built-in wash down facilities.
C) Construction should allow for easy visual inspection.
D) Utility controls should be inside the hood.

11) Which statement best characterizes the implication of substituting the term "design to achieve minimum risk" with the term "design to achieve acceptable risk"?

A) The two terms are synonymous.
B) Designing to achieve acceptable risk is appropriate only when designing to achieve minimum risk is shown to be unachievable.
C) Designing to achieve minimum risk may require spending much more money to reduce the risk of a certain event far below what would be an acceptable risk level.
D) Designing to achieve minimum risk is what safety and health professionals should solely advocate since they must have no opinion on what constitutes acceptable risk.

12) A __________ is an object that connects a piece of electrical equipment to earth or some conducting body that serves in place of earth.

A) Bond.
B) Ground.
C) Metal frame.
D) Double-insulation.

13) Damaged electrical equipment:

A) Should be removed from service.
B) Indicates a lack of supervisory accountability.
C) Indicates unsafe employee behavior.
D) Indicates a lack of safety resources.

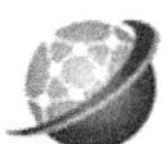

14) Only a small percentage of car accidents are the result of mechanical failure. How can a company **best** control the major cause driver error?
  A) Conducting monthly safety meetings.
  B) Requiring substance abuse testing of all drivers.
  C) Hiring only drivers under 40 years of age.
  D) Implementing a program of driver selection, training and supervisor observation.

15) A canopy hood **would not** be considered an acceptable ventilation system for a large solvent dip tank if:
  A) The hood would be unacceptably large.
  B) Larger fans are needed.
  C) Contaminant is drawn through breathing zone.
  D) A hood would get in the way of the lifting device.

16) The **final** step in a machine lockout procedure is to:
  A) Verbally announce that the machine is now locked-out.
  B) Release all stored or residual energy sources.
  C) Verify the isolation of the equipment by operating the machine controls.
  D) Make sure all emergency stop buttons have been depressed.

17) Tag attachments must warn employees about machine hazards if energized and be standardized, self-locking, non-releasable, with a **minimum** unlocking strength of
  A) 50 lbs.
  B) 25 lbs.
  C) 10 lbs.
  D) 75 lbs.

18) During an inspection of an industrial area you observe an operator being sprayed by fluids from the process. Which control recommendation to management is the **best?**
  A) Determine the exposure limits for the fluids.
  B) Instruct the worker to report any skin irritations.
  C) Design a splash shield to protect the operator.
  D) Provide PPE and train the worker to avoid splashes.

19) Chemical hazards are generally divided into the following categories:
    A) Toxic, reactive, corrosive, and flammable.
    B) Toxic, reactive, acids, and combustibles.
    C) Inert, organic, hydrocarbons and cryogens.
    D) Acids, bases, explosives and hydrocarbons.

20) Verification that the procedures and practices developed under the Process Safety Management standard are adequate requires certification of compliance every:
    A) 5 years.
    B) 3 years.
    C) Annually.
    D) Based on company compliance.

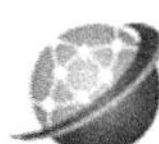

Domain 3 Quiz 2 Answers

1) Answer C:

Safety through design is defined as the integration of hazard analysis and risk assessment methods early in the design and redesign processes and taking the actions necessary so that the risks of injury or damage are at an acceptable level. This concept encompasses facilities, hardware, equipment, tools, materials, layout and configuration, energy controls, environmental concerns and products.

- **Severity is** the extent of harm or damage that could result from an incident.
- **Prevention through design is** addressing occupational safety and health needs in design and redesign processes to prevent or minimize work-related hazards and risks associated with the construction, manufacture, use, maintenance, and disposal of facilities, materials, equipment and processes.
- **Hierarchy of controls is a** systematic way of thinking and acting, considering steps in a ranked and sequential order, to choose the most effective means of eliminating or reducing hazards and the risks that derive from them.

An example is the requirement of suppliers of services to attest that processes have been applied to identify and analyze hazards and to reduce the risks deriving from those hazards to an acceptable level.

[There is precedent for having suppliers attest that risk analyses have been completed. Manufacturers of equipment to be used in the European Union are required by International Organization for Standardization (ISO) standards to certify that they have met applicable standards, including ISO 12100-1 and ISO 14121.]

2) Answer C:

As per the OSHA 1910.146 Standard,

"Confined space" means a space that:

(1) Is large enough and so configured that an employee can bodily enter and perform assigned work; and

(2) Has limited or restricted means for entry or exit (for example, tanks, vessels, silos, storage bins, hoppers, vaults, and pits are spaces that may have limited means of entry.); and

(3) Is not designed for continuous employee occupancy.

"Non-permit confined space" means a confined space that does not contain or, with respect to atmospheric hazards, have the potential to contain any hazard capable of causing death or serious physical harm. **"Permit-required confined space (permit space)"** means a confined space that has one or more of the following characteristics:

(1) Contains or has a potential to contain a hazardous atmosphere;

(2) Contains a material that has the potential for engulfing an entrant;

(3) Has an internal configuration such that an entrant could be trapped or asphyxiated by inwardly converging walls or by a floor which slopes downward and tapers to a smaller cross-section; or

(4) Contains any other recognized serious safety or health hazard.

"Permit-required confined space program (permit space program)" means the employer's overall program for controlling, and, where appropriate, for protecting employees from, permit space hazards and for regulating employee entry into permit spaces. "Entry permit (permit)" means the written or printed document that is provided by the employer to allow and control entry into a permit space. "Permit system" means the employer's written procedure for preparing and issuing permits for entry and for returning the permit space to service following termination of entry.

3) Answer A:

"Isolation" means the process by which a permit space is removed from service and completely protected against the release of energy and material into the space by such means as: blanking or blinding; misaligning or removing sections of lines, pipes, or ducts; a double block and bleed system; lockout or tagout of all sources of energy; or blocking or disconnecting all mechanical linkages.

"Double block and bleed" means the closure of a line, duct, or pipe by closing and locking or tagging two in-line valves and by opening and locking or tagging a drain or vent valve in the line between the two closed valves.

"Blanking or blinding" means the absolute closure of a pipe, line, or duct by the fastening of a solid plate (such as a spectacle blind or a skillet blind) that completely covers the bore and that is capable of withstanding the maximum pressure of the pipe, line, or duct with no leakage beyond the plate.

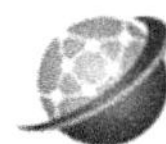

"Line breaking" means the intentional opening of a pipe, line, or duct that is or has been carrying flammable, corrosive, or toxic material, an inert gas, or any fluid at a volume, pressure, or temperature capable of causing injury.

"Inerting" means the displacement of the atmosphere in a permit space by a noncombustible gas (such as nitrogen) to such an extent that the resulting atmosphere is noncombustible. *NOTE:* This procedure produces an IDLH oxygen-deficient atmosphere.

4) Answer C:

Atmospheric testing is required for two distinct purposes: evaluation of the hazards of the permit space and verification that acceptable conditions exist for entry into that space. Verification testing is done to make sure that the chemical hazards that may be present are below the levels necessary for safe entry, and that they meet the conditions identified on the permit. Test the atmosphere in the following order: (1) for oxygen, (2) for combustible gases, and then (3) for toxic gases and vapors. The testing results, the actual test concentrations, must be recorded on the permit near the levels identified for safe entry. The testing results and the decisions about what steps must be followed before entry must be evaluated by, or reviewed by, a technically qualified professional like, a certified industrial hygienist, a registered safety engineer, or a certified safety professional. The technically qualified professional must consider all of the serious hazards in his/her evaluation or review. Code of Federal Regulations 1910.146, Appendix B.

"Hazardous atmosphere" means an atmosphere that may expose employees to the risk of death, incapacitation, and impairment of ability to self-rescue (that is, escape unaided from a permit space), injury, or acute illness from one or more of the following causes:

(1) Flammable gas, vapor, or mist in excess of 10 percent of its lower flammable limit (LFL);

(2) Airborne combustible dust at a concentration that meets or exceeds its LFL; *NOTE:* This concentration may be approximated as a condition in which the **dust obscures vision at a distance of 5 feet** (1.52 m) or less.

(3) Atmospheric oxygen concentration below 19.5 percent or above 23.5 percent;

(4) Atmospheric concentration of any substance for which a dose or a permissible exposure limit is published in Subpart G, Occupational Health and Environmental Control, or in Subpart Z, Toxic and Hazardous Substances, of this Part and which could result in employee exposure in excess of its dose or permissible exposure limit; *NOTE:* An atmospheric concentration of any substance that is not capable of causing death, incapacitation, and impairment

of ability to self-rescue, injury, or acute illness due to its health effects is not covered by this provision.
(5) Any other atmospheric condition that is immediately dangerous to life or health. Code of Federal Regulations 1910.146, Appendix A

5) Answer C:
Infrared radiation has wavelengths from 700nm to 1mm and is characterized by smaller bands. IR-A (near infrared) is the spectral region from 701 to 1400 nm. IR-B includes wavelengths from 1.4 to 100mm. The IR-C spectrum is 0.1 to 1 mm. Most radiative heat transfer involves the infrared region. Sources of infrared typically are sources of radiative heat, including fires and open flames, stoves, electrical heating elements, certain lasers, and many other sources. Near infrared radiation (700–1400 nm) passes through the lens of the eye to the retina or is refracted from other tissues. High energy levels can cause a variety of eye disorders, among which is scotoma. Scotoma is loss of vision in a portion of the visual field resulting from damage to the retina where radiation is absorbed. Other disorders range from simple reddening from low-level exposures to swelling of the eye, hemorrhaging, and lesions. Extended exposures to infrared radiation can cause cataracts. Common examples are glassblower's and bottlemaker's cataracts that result from looking into fire and heat sources. Iron workers who peer into furnaces extensively have a high incidence of cataracts. To limit the danger from infrared radiation, limit the duration of exposure and the intensity of exposure. Because the danger is mainly to the retina of the eye, looking into infrared sources should be avoided. The intensity of exposure is most easily reduced by shielding. Eyewear that absorbs and reduces the amount of infrared reaching the eye should be worn. Lenses in glasses, goggles, or faceshields must have the correct shade to reduce harmful levels. (Brauer, 2006)

6) Answer A:
There are three traditional levels of warnings:

- Danger is used where there is an immediate hazard, which, if encountered, will result in severe personal injury or death.
- Warning is the signal word for hazards or unsafe practices which could result in severe personal injury or death.
- Caution is used for hazards or unsafe practices which could usually result in minor personal injury, product damage, or property damage.

Evaluation of the warning adequacy at minimum requires consideration the dangerousness of the product, the intensity of and form of the warning given, the likelihood that a particular warning will be adequately communicated. The burden is upon the manufacturer to provide such

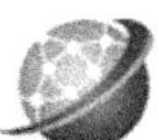

warnings.

7) Answer C:
The word "sign" refers to a surface on prepared for the warning of, or safety instructions of, industrial workers or members of the public who may be exposed to hazards. Excluded from this definition, however, are news releases, displays commonly known as safety posters, and bulletins used for employee education.
The wording of any sign should be easily read and concise. The sign should contain sufficient information to be easily understood. The wording should make a positive, rather than negative suggestion and should be accurate in fact.
"Major message" means that portion of a tag's inscription that is more specific than the signal word and that indicates the specific hazardous condition or an instruction to be communicated to the employee. Examples include: "High Voltage," "Close Clearance," "Do Not Start," or "Do Not Use" or a corresponding pictograph used with a written text or alone.
"Signal word" means that portion of a tag's inscription that contains the word or words that are intended to capture the employee's immediate attention.

8) Answer D:
Proof test is a nondestructive tension test performed by the sling manufacturer or an equivalent entity to verify construction and workmanship of a sling. The proof testing of slings is the responsibility of the sling manufacturer or equivalent entity as delineated by the standard at 29 CFR 1910.184(e)(4), (g)(5), and (i)(8)(ii). The employer shall retain a "certificate of proof test"

9) Answer D:
When working with a combustion heater in an enclosed workspace, carbon monoxide is a concern. A continuous supply fresh air flow is needed for proper air changes to reduce the buildup of Carbon Monoxide (CO).

10) Answer D:

The greatest concern would be operator controls located inside the hood. Never use perchloric acid in a hood designed for other purposes. Perchloric acid $HClO_4$ is a common acid used primarily by the chemical, electroplating and incendiary (fireworks) industries. It is a strong oxidizing acid that reacts with organic compounds, including cellulosic materials such as sawdust and cork. A mixture of perchloric acid and these materials may ignite spontaneously. Therefore, hoods and ducts must be nonreactive, easily cleaned and inspected for acid build-up, and should include water wash-down capability. The ACGIH Industrial Ventilation Manual contains a list of design and work practices for perchloric acid hoods. They recommend stainless steel with rounded corners and all-welded construction.

11) Answer C:

Those who oppose the use of the term acceptable risk often offer substitute terms. One frequent suggestion is to say that designers and operators should achieve *minimum* risk levels or *minimize* the risks. Requiring that systems be designed and operated to minimum risk levels, that risks be minimized, is impractical because the investments necessary to do so may be so high that the cost of the product required to recoup the investment and make a reasonable profit would not be competitive in the marketplace.

12) Answer B:

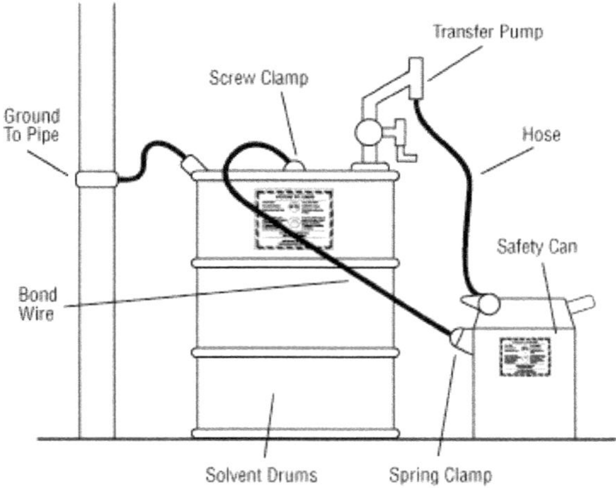

This is the definition of a ground and a bond according to the NSC. The continuity test ensures that the equipment grounding conductor is electrically continuous.

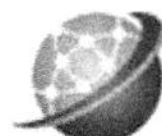

13) Answer A:
Defective electrical equipment that might expose an employee to injury should be removed from service. (Haight, 2012)

14) Answer D:
According to the NSC, "Companies can control driver error by introducing a program of driver selection, training and supervision, while vehicle failure can be reduced by implementing a preventive maintenance program."

15) Answer C:
Since canopies are above the worker the contaminant must travel very close to, and most of the time through, the worker's breathing zone.

16) Answer C:
"Lockout/tagout" refers to specific practices and procedures to safeguard employees from the unexpected energization or startup of machinery and equipment, or the release of hazardous energy during service or maintenance activities.1 This requires, in part, that a designated individual turns off and disconnects the machinery or equipment from its energy source(s) before performing service or maintenance and that the authorized employee(s) either lock or tag the energy-isolating device(s) to prevent the release of hazardous energy and take steps to verify that the energy has been isolated effectively. If the potential exists for the release of hazardous stored energy or for the reaccumulation of stored energy to a hazardous level, the employer must ensure that the employee(s) take steps to prevent injury that may result from the release of the stored energy.

Lockout devices hold energy-isolation devices in a safe or "off" position. They provide protection by preventing machines or equipment from becoming energized because they are positive restraints that no one can remove without a key or other unlocking mechanism, or through extraordinary means, such as bolt cutters. Tagout devices, by contrast, are prominent warning devices that an authorized employee fastens to energy-isolating devices to warn employees not to reenergize the machine while he or she services or maintains it. Tagout devices are easier to remove and, by themselves, provide employees with less protection than do lockout devices. As part of an energy-control program, employers must:

- Establish energy-control procedures for removing the energy supply from machines and for putting appropriate lockout or tagout devices on the energy-isolating devices to prevent unexpected re-energization. When appropriate, the procedure also must address stored or potentially re-accumulated energy;
- Train employees on the energy-control program, including the safe application, use, and removal of energy controls; and
- Inspect these procedures periodically (at least annually) to ensure that they are being followed and that they remain effective in preventing employee exposure to hazardous energy.

In Appendix A to 1910.147, OSHA provides a *Typical Minimal Lockout Procedur*e Before beginning service or maintenance, the following steps must be accomplished in sequence and according to the specific provisions of the employer's energy-control procedure:

1. Prepare for shutdown;
2. Shut down the machine;
3. Disconnect or isolate the machine from the energy source(s);
4. Apply the lockout or tagout device(s) to the energy-isolating device(s);
5. Release, restrain, or otherwise render safe all potential hazardous stored or residual energy. If a possibility exists for reaccumulation of hazardous energy, regularly verify during the service and maintenance that such energy has not reaccumulated to hazardous levels; and
6. Verify the isolation and deenergization of the machine.
7. (OSHA Publication 3120, 2002)

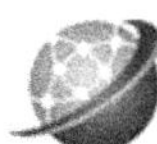

17) Answer A:

A tagout device is a prominent warning that clearly states that the machinery being controlled must not be operated until the tag is removed in accordance with an established procedure. Tags are essentially warning devices and do not provide the physical restraint of a lock. Tags may evoke a false sense of security. For these reasons, OSHA considers lockout devices to be more secure and more effective than tagout devices in protecting employees from hazardous energy. Whether lockout or tagout devices are used, they must be the only devices the employer uses in conjunction with energy-isolating devices to control hazardous energy. The employer must provide these devices and they must be singularly identified and not used for other purposes. In addition, they must have the following characteristics:

- Durable enough to withstand workplace conditions. Tagout devices must not deteriorate or become illegible even when used with corrosive components such as acid or alkali chemicals or in wet environments.
- Standardized according to color, shape, or size. Tagout devices also must be standardized according to print and format. Tags must be legible and understandable by all employees. They must warn employees about the hazards if the machine is energized, and offer employees clear instruction such as: "Do Not Start,"
- Substantial enough to minimize the likelihood of premature or accidental removal. Employees should be able to remove locks only by using excessive force with special tools such as bolt cutters or other metal-cutting tools. Tag attachments must be non-reusable, self-locking, and non-releasable, with a **minimum unlocking strength of 50 pounds**. Tags must be attachable by hand, and the device for attaching the tag should be a one-piece nylon cable tie or its equivalent so it can withstand all environments and conditions.
- Labeled to identify the specific employees authorized to apply and remove them.

Training must ensure that employees understand the purpose, function, and restrictions of the energy-control program. Employers must provide training specific to the needs of "authorized," "affected," and "other" employees.

"Authorized" employees are those responsible for implementing the energy-control procedures or performing the service or maintenance activities. They need the knowledge and skills necessary for the safe application, use, and removal of energy-isolating devices. They also need training in the following:

- Hazardous energy source recognition;
- The type and magnitude of the hazardous energy sources in the workplace; and
- Energy-control procedures, including the methods and means to isolate and control those energy sources.

"Affected" employees (usually machine operators or users) are employees who operate the relevant machinery or whose jobs require them to be in the area where service or maintenance is performed. These employees do not service or maintain machinery or perform lockout/tagout activities. Affected employees must receive training in the purpose and use of energy-control procedures. They also need to be able to do the following:

- Recognize when the energy-control procedure is being used,
- Understand the purpose of the procedure, and
- Understand the importance of not tampering with lockout or tagout devices and not starting or using equipment that has been locked or tagged out.

The employer must provide initial training before starting service and maintenance activities and must provide retraining as necessary. In addition, the employer must certify that the training has been given provided.

18) Answer C:

The best solution is to prevent worker exposure to the fluids. Splash shields and enclosures are examples of engineering controls designed to protect the worker from splash hazards.

19) Answer A:

Chemical hazards are generally divided into toxic, reactive, corrosive, and flammable subcategories. Hazardous waste is characterized by toxicity, corrosivity, ignitability, and reactivity.

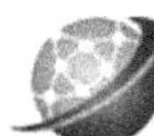

20) Answer B:

According to OSHA Publication 3132 Process Safety Management:

- Employers shall certify that they have evaluated compliance with the provisions of the PSM standard at least every three years to verify that the procedures and practices developed under the standard are adequate are being followed. The compliance audit must be conducted by at least one person knowledgeable in the process and a report of the findings of the audit must be developed and documented noting deficiencies that have been corrected. The two most recent compliance audit reports must be kept on file.
- All process hazard analyses must be updated and revalidated, based on their completion date, at least every five (5) years. The process hazard analysis shall be performed by a team with expertise in engineering and process operations, and the team shall include at least one employee who has experience and knowledge specific to the process being evaluated. Also, one member of the team must be knowledgeable in the specific process hazard analysis methodology being used.
- Incident investigation reports must be retained for five years and must be initiated as promptly as possible, but not later than 48 hours following the incident.
- Inspection and testing must be performed on process equipment, using procedures that follow recognized and generally accepted good engineering practices. The frequency of inspections and tests of process equipment must conform to manufacturers' recommendations and good engineering practices, or more frequently if determined to be necessary by prior operating experience. Each inspection and test on process equipment must be documented, identifying the date of the inspection or test, the name of the person who performed the inspection or test, the serial number or other identifier of the equipment on which the inspection or test was performed, a description of the inspection or test performed, and the results of the inspection or test.
- Training must include emphasis on the specific safety and health hazards of the process, emergency operations including shutdown, and other safe work practices that apply to the employee's job tasks. Refresher training must be provided at least every three years. The employer must determine whether each employee operating a process has received and understood the training required by PSM. A record must be kept containing the identity of the employee, the date of training, and how the employer verified that the employee understood the training.

Domain 3 Quiz 3 Questions

1) The movement of liquids or vapors through a garment material that occurs on a molecular level is called:
   A) Penetration.
   B) Osmosis.
   C) Convection.
   D) Permeation.

2) There is a process in an industrial operation that utilizes vinyl chloride. The concentration in the operational area is 400 ppm. The **best** respiratory protection at this exposure level is
   A) APR with HEPA filter.
   B) half-face SAR.
   C) full-face SAR in negative mode with escape bottle.
   D) positive pressure SCBA.

3) Spoiling evidence would include:
   A) Loss of evidence.
   B) Destruction of evidence.
   C) Tampering with evidence.
   D) Chain of custody.

4) Monthly fire extinguisher checks involve proper extinguisher type, mounting, accessibility, gauge pressure and
   A) Annual inspection tag, signs of corrosion.
   B) Perform hydro static testing, name plate.
   C) Safety pin, handle squeeze.
   D) Nozzle, internal tube.

5) Operation is grinding and workers using full face respirators with a combination cartridge of vapor/organic vapor are they protected?
   A) No, a particulate respirator is needed.
   B) No, respirators are not required for grinding operations.
   C) Yes, combinations cartridges are acceptable.
   D) Yes, organic vapor cartridges will filter particulates.

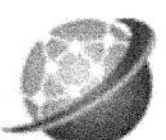

6) An example of an unsafe act is:
   A) Flammable atmosphere in a confined space.
   B) Failing to properly secure a load picked from a flatbed trailer.
   C) Broken scaffolding plank within two feet from the cross brace.
   D) Fall protection anchor points not available.

7) Which of the following statements is **most** correct concerning electrical Ground Fault Circuit Interrupters (GFCI)?
   A) GFCIs will trip at about 7-9 milliamps leakage line-to-line fault current.
   B) GFCIs will trip at about 1-3 milliamps leakage line-to-ground fault current.
   C) GFCIs will protect against leakage line to ground and line to line faults and trip at about 15-20 amperes.
   D) GFCIs will trip at about 4-6 milliamps leakage line-to-ground fault current.

8) The conditions **most** common to crane side loading are:
   A) High wind, "OFF rubber", boom extended.
   B) load is dragged, not level, high wind.
   C) hook on center of load, shock loading, outriggers set.
   D) not level, high wind, "ON rubber".

9) Best practices in Environmental Management-Spill Response include planning, personal protective equipment, mitigation and:
   A) Decontamination.
   B) Litigation.
   C) Spill accountability.
   D) Restoration.

10) The employee working in an area where asbestos could be disturbed is entitled to:
   A) A copy of the SDS for asbestos and chest X-rays.
   B) Information about ACM or PACM only in occupied buildings older than 1980.
   C) Training, as provided for all exposed employees working in the area or could disturb asbestos.
   D) Work without respiratory protection when wet methods are not used, and asbestos is friable.

11) Which reason is frequently associated with hazardous material releases from underground storage tanks?
   A) Tampering.
   B) Piping failure.
   C) Soil subsidence.
   D) Thermal shock.

12) The certification process offers a certification process for new building construction and renovations which includes a rating system, designed to guide and distinguish high performance buildings that have **less** of an impact on the environment and are healthier to work within is called:
   A) GREEN.
   B) ALARA.
   C) LEED.
   D) ASHARE.

13) Best protection for working long durations in a permit required confined space with monitoring readings of 14% O_2 and CO 500 ppm is a:
   A) Supplied air respirator with escape bottle.
   B) SCBA in negative pressure mode.
   C) Powered APR with organic vapor cartridge in negative pressure mode.
   D) Air purifying respirator with HEPA filtration.

14) An SMS is evaluating worker radon exposure in an Ozarks underground laboratory. The **primary** concern with long term exposure to radon gas is:
   A) Dermatitis and skin sensitization.
   B) Increased risk of lung cancer.
   C) Eye irritation and cataracts.
   D) Gastrointestinal and liver disease.

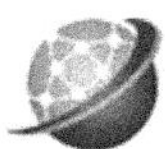

15) Environmental management guidelines are generally composed of a series of interlinking and supporting components which include:
   A) A set of principles, tools to achieve environmental objectives, management programs, a management framework.
   B) A set of regulatory standards, tools to achieve environmental objectives, management programs, a management framework.
   C) A set of principles, tools to achieve environmental objectives, management programs.
   D) A set of regulatory standards, tools to achieve environmental objectives, a management framework.

16) What are the colors on a corrosive placard?
   A) Red, Yellow.
   B) Red, White.
   C) Black, White.
   D) Yellow, Black.

17) The **most** important factor of wrench design is:
   A) The purpose of the tool and how it will be used.
   B) The type of metals used and grip strength.
   C) The type of worker and work environment.
   D) The use of self-opening springs and grip size.

18) What is the **best** solution to protect for workers exposed to noise for 4 hours at 115 dBA?
   A) Attenuate exposure to a protected TWA of 95 dBA.
   B) Reduce the noise from the source.
   C) Limit the work time of exposure to two hours.
   D) Provide appropriate hearing protection.

19) Which of the following are prioritized from **most effective** to **least effective**?

A) Substitution, Elimination, engineering controls, warnings, administrative controls, personal protective equipment.
B) Elimination, engineering controls, substitution, administrative controls, warnings, personal protective equipment.
C) Engineering controls, Elimination, substitution, administrative controls, warnings, personal protective equipment.
D) Elimination, substitution, engineering controls, warnings, administrative controls, personal protective equipment.

20) To protect unqualified workers from arc flash hazards, at what boundary should nonconductive barriers should be placed?

A) Shock protection boundary.
B) Restricted approach boundary.
C) Limited approach boundary.
D) Prohibited approach boundary.

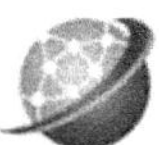

Domain 3 Quiz 3 Answers

1) Answer D:

Permeation involves sorption of the chemical into the surface of the material, diffusion through the material, and desorption on the opposite side.
Osmosis is a process by which molecules of a solvent tend to pass through a semipermeable membrane from a less concentrated solution into a more concentrated one, thus equalizing the concentrations on each side of the membrane
Convection is the movement caused within a fluid (gas or liquid) by the tendency of hotter and therefore less dense material to rise, and colder, denser material to sink under the influence of gravity, which consequently results in transfer of heat.
Penetration is the passage of vapors or liquids through zippers, seams, holes, etc
Degradation is the physical changes to the material caused by the chemical, which can include swelling, stiffening, wrinkling, changes in color, and other physical deterioration.

2) Answer D:

Vinyl chloride is a suspected carcinogen with an OSHA TWA of 1 ppm (ACGIH TLV 5 ppm) for 8 hours and a 15 minute ceiling limit of 5 ppm. NIOSH recommends respiratory protection to consist of self-contained breathing apparatus with full-face piece and operated in a positive-pressure mode. A full-face respirator with airline can be utilized if operated in positive-pressure mode and used in combination with an auxiliary self-contained breathing apparatus operated in a positive-pressure mode. A full-face respirator operated in a positive-pressure mode provides a protection factor of "1000", **while an SCBA provides a protection factor of approximately "10,000"**.

Assigned Protection Factors					
Type of Respirator	**Quarter mask**	**Half mask**	**Full facepiece**	**Helmet/Hood**	**Loose-fitting facepiece**
1. Air-Purifying Respirator	5	10	50	—	—
2. Powered Air-Purifying Respirator (PAPR)	—	50	1,000	25/1,000	25
Supplied-Air Respirator (SAR) or Airline Respirator					
• Demand mode	—	10	50	— 25/1,000	— 25
• Continuous flow mode	—	50	1,000	—	—
• Pressure-demand or other positive-pressure mode	—	50	1,000		
Self-Contained Breathing Apparatus (SCBA)					
• Demand mode	—	10	50	50	—
• Pressure-demand or other positive- pressure mode (e.g., open/closed circuit)—	—	—	10,000	10,000	—
OSHA 3352-02 2009 Assigned Protection Factors for the Revised Respiratory Protection Standard.					

The Maximum use concentration (MUC) for respirators is calculated by multiplying the APF for the respirator by the PEL. The MUC is the upper limit at which the class of respirator is expected to provide protection.

MUC = TLV x APF

End-of-service-life indicator (ESLI) means a system that warns the respirator user of the approach of the end of adequate respiratory protection, for example, that the sorbent is approaching saturation or is no longer effective.

3) Answer C:

The **spoliation of evidence** is the intentional, reckless, or negligent withholding, hiding, altering, fabricating, or destroying of evidence relevant to a legal proceeding. Chain of custody is documentation of possession.

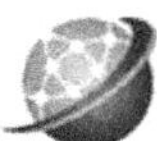

4) Answer A:

To prevent fire extinguishers from being moved or damaged, they should be mounted on brackets or in wall cabinets with the carrying handle placed 3-1/2 to 5 feet above the floor. Larger fire extinguishers need to be mounted at lower heights with the carrying handle about 3 feet from the floor. Portable extinguishers shall be visually inspected monthly to verify:

- Is each extinguisher in its designated place, clearly visible, and not blocked by equipment, coats or other objects that could interfere with access during an emergency?
- Is the nameplate with operating instructions legible and facing outward?
- Is the pressure gauge showing that the extinguisher is fully charged (the needle should be in the green zone)?
- Is the pin and tamper seal intact?
- Is the extinguisher in good condition and showing no signs of physical damage, corrosion, or leakage?
- Have all dry powder extinguishers been gently rocked top to bottom to make sure the powder is not packing?

OSHA 1910.157 requires that portable fire extinguishers are hydrostatically tested whenever they show new evidence of corrosion or mechanical injury. The employer shall assure that portable fire extinguishers are subjected to an annual maintenance check. Stored pressure extinguishers do not require an internal examination. The employer shall record the annual maintenance date and retain this record for one year after the last entry or the life of the shell, whichever is less. Where the employer has provided portable fire extinguishers for employee use in the workplace, the employer shall also provide an educational program to familiarize employees with the general principles of fire extinguisher use and the hazards involved with incipient stage fire fighting

5) Answer A:

Grinding operations can produce dust particles and would require a particulate respirator.

Particulate Respirators

- Capture particles in the air, such as dusts, mists, and fumes.
- Do not protect against gases or vapors.
- Generally become more effective as particles accumulate on the filter and plug spaces between the fibers.
- Filters should be replaced when user finds it difficult to breathe through them.

Combination Respirators

- Are normally used in atmospheres that contain hazards of both particulates and gases.
- Have both particulate filters and gas/vapor filters.
- May be heavier.

Gas & Vapor Respirators

- Are normally used when there are only hazardous gases and vapors in the air.
- Use chemical filters (called cartridges or canisters) to remove dangerous gases or vapors.
- Do not protect against airborne particles.
- Are made to protect against specific gases or vapors.
- Provide protection only as long as the filter's absorbing capacity is not depleted.
- The service life of the filter depends upon many factors and can be estimated in various ways.

6) Answer B:

Heinrich's Domino Theory states that accidents result from a chain of sequential events, metaphorically like a line of dominoes falling over. When one of the dominoes falls, it triggers the next one, and the next...but removing a key factor (such as an unsafe condition or an unsafe act) prevents the start of the chain reaction. According to Heinrich, all incidents directly relate to unsafe conditions and acts. Unsafe acts could involve unsafe performance of persons, such as standing under suspended loads, failing to properly secure a load, horseplay, and removal of safeguards. Unsafe conditions could include environmental chemical hazards such as a confined space atmosphere, mechanical or physical hazards such as unguarded gears and insufficient light.

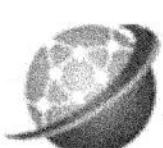

7) Answer D:

The range of 70-100 mA is widely accepted as enough current to produce a fatality. The ground-fault circuit interrupter (GFCI) is a fast acting device, when even a small amount of current (about 5 milliamp) passes to ground any path other than the proper conductor and in a fraction of a second shuts off the power to the circuit. The GFCI will not sense a line-to-line fault. Construction sites must guard against ground faults either by installing GFCIs or through an assured equipment grounding conductor program. To provide the best protection, use GFCIs on all 120 and 240 volt receptacles. Placed between the electrical service and the tool or appliance it serves, the GFCI continually monitors the amount of current going to and from the tool along the normal path of the circuit conductors. Whenever the amount *going* differs from the amount *returning* by a set trip level the GFCI interrupts the electric power within 1/40th of a second. This difference in current is called leakage current to ground and the path it takes to ground could be through a person - in which case, the rapid response of the GFCI is fast enough to prevent electrocution. This protection provided by the GFCI is independent of the condition of the equipment grounding conductor, thus, the GFCI can provide protection even if the equipment grounding conductor becomes inoperative. However, it will not detect line-to-line faults.

8) Answer B:

The load chart ratings apply only to freely suspended loads and when the load is picked up directly under the boom tip. If the load is to either side of the boom tip, side loading occurs, which affects the crane's capacity. Side loading is one of the most common causes of boom failure and usually occurs without warning. Side loading can occur when a load is dragged or pulled sideways, when the load starts swinging rapidly, when the crane is not level, and when exposed to high wind speeds. Tilt-up construction methods can also cause side loading of the boom. Shock loading can be caused by rapid acceleration, sudden stopping, sudden load release, and sudden load snatching.

The key to lifting a maximum capacity load with a mobile crane is the outriggers. They provide a solid platform for the crane's safe operation and efficient use. Operators and workers within a crane's radius must always be aware of how critical the placement and use of outriggers are to the crane's performance. Statistics show that at least 50% of crane incidents occur because the mobile crane or outriggers are not set-up properly. Specific hazards that can cause or contribute to failure or collapse include:

- failure to extend the outriggers fully;
- not extending all outriggers;

- failure to get completely "off-rubber"
- not accounting for poor ground conditions;
- failure to level the crane

Use the Correct Load Chart: The purpose of outriggers is to improve the stability of the crane. Accurate use of the *"on-outriggers fully extended"* load chart, requires that outriggers be fully extended, and they must bring the rig completely off-rubber. If the tires are touching the ground, then the *"on-rubber"* load chart is the only one that can be used. Manufacturers do not recommend extending only one or two of the outriggers. If outriggers are to be used, fully extend all of them and get the tires off the ground. Accidents commonly occur because the operator is lifting from only one side of the rig, with only two outriggers extended. Then, later in the day, this same operator is asked to swing the boom to the other side of the rig for a pick. He does this without thinking and topples the crane. Outrigger Pads and Floats: The pads found on all crane outriggers are designed for good ground conditions. Poor conditions reduce the amount of load a crane can safely place on the outrigger pad. Because of this, many crane operations require additional support or "floats." Supplemental floats are made of substantial material and must *always* be larger than the outrigger pad. These floats disperse the weight of the crane and its load over more ground area than does the pad. Any float or cribbing which is smaller than the pad, increases the pressure placed on the ground. This increase in pressure, particularly in poor ground conditions, can cause an outrigger to "punch through," and bring about an accident. Leveling: Also be aware that all floats and cribbing must be level. If the outrigger pad is set down on an unleveled float, the outrigger pad may slide off when under load, causing the crane to tip. Many manufacturers stipulate that the crane must be within 1% of level before their load chart applies.

9) Answer A:

Industry best practices incorporate incident planning, written plans, and practice exercises as essential elements of a successful emergency response. Best practices include general concepts such as planning, PPE, mitigation, and decontamination, but these must be adapted to provide for any site-specific conditions and contingencies.

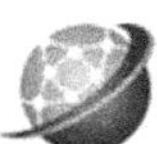

10) Answer C:

According to OSHA 29 CFR 1910.1001, the employer shall institute a training program

- For all employees who are exposed to airborne concentrations of asbestos at or above the PEL and/or excursion limit and ensure their participation in the program.
- Training shall be provided prior to or at the time of initial assignment and at least annually thereafter.
- The employer shall also provide, at no cost to employees who perform housekeeping operations in an area which contains ACM or PACM, an asbestos awareness training course, which shall at a minimum contain the following elements: health effects of asbestos, locations of ACM and PACM in the building/facility, recognition of ACM and PACM damage and deterioration, requirements in this standard relating to housekeeping, and proper response to fiber release episodes, to all employees who perform housekeeping work in areas where ACM and/or PACM is present.
- Each such employee shall be so trained at least once a year.

The OSHA standard establishes a classification system for asbestos construction work that spells out mandatory, simple, technological work practices that employers must follow to reduce worker exposures. Under this system, the following four classes of construction work are matched with increasingly stringent control requirements:

- ***Class I*** asbestos work is the most potentially hazardous class of asbestos jobs. This work involves the removal of asbestos-containing thermal system insulation and sprayed-on or troweled-on surfacing materials. Employers must presume that thermal system insulation and surfacing material found in pre-1981 construction is ACM. That presumption, however, is rebuttable. If you believe that the surfacing material or thermal system insulation is not ACM, the OSHA standard specifies the means that you must use to rebut that presumption. Thermal system insulation includes ACM applied to pipes, boilers, tanks, ducts, or other structural components to prevent heat loss or gain. Surfacing materials include decorative plaster on ceilings and walls; acoustical materials on decking, walls, and ceilings; and fireproofing on structural members.
- ***Class II*** work includes the removal of other types of ACM that are not thermal system insulation such as resilient flooring and roofing materials. Examples of Class II work include removal of asbestos-containing floor or ceiling tiles, siding, roofing, or transite panels.
- ***Class III*** asbestos work includes repair and maintenance operations where ACM or presumed ACM (PACM) are disturbed.
- ***Class IV*** work includes custodial activities where employees clean up asbestos-

containing waste and debris produced by construction, maintenance, or repair activities. This work involves cleaning dust-contaminated surfaces, vacuuming contaminated carpets, mopping floors, and cleaning up ACM or PACM from thermal system insulation or surfacing material.

Some people exposed to asbestos in industrial environment have developed a cancer called *mesothelioma*. Mesothelioma affects mesothelial tissue used by the body for linings or sacs. These linings/sacs are found in the body's pulmonary and abdominal cavities. Persons known to develop these types of cancers include insulation workers who inhale gross amounts of asbestos, especially *chrysotile*.

11) Answer B:

According to EPA studies, the releases from underground storage tanks (USTs) are typically associated with these problems: (1) piping failure, (2) corrosion, (3) spills and overfilling.

12) Answer C:

Many organizations have found that undertaking a serious pollution prevention effort is a successful business response because it reduces their regulatory burden, increases public confidence, reduces long term risk, and nearly always cuts costs. Designed primarily for new construction office buildings, the ***Leadership in Energy and Environmental Design (LEED)*** certification process has been applied to many other commercial building types. LEED certification is a performance-oriented rating system where building projects earn points for satisfying criterion designed to address specific environmental impacts inherent in the design, construction, operations and management of a building. The LEED certification system is organized into six environmental categories: Sustainable Sites, Water Efficiency, Energy and Atmosphere, Materials and Resources, Indoor Environmental Quality and Innovation & Design.

13) Answer A:

A supplied air respirator with an escape bottle with be the best selection for confined space operations with potentially oxygen deficient or toxic hazardous atmospheres. Respirators protect the user in two basic ways. The first is by the removal of contaminants from the air. Respirators of this type include particulate respirators, which filter out airborne particles, and air-purifying respirators with cartridges/canisters which filter out chemicals and gases. Other respirators protect by supplying clean respirable air from another source. Respirators that fall into this

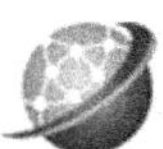

category include airline respirators, which use compressed air from a remote source, and self-contained breathing apparatus (SCBA), which include their own air supply.

Hazard	**Respirator**
Immediately dangerous to life or health (IDLH)	
Oxygen deficiency Gas, vapor contaminants and other highly toxic air contaminants	Full-facepiece, pressure-demand SCBA certified for a minimum service life of 30 minutes. A combination full-facepiece, pressure-demand SAR with an auxiliary self-contained air supply.
Contaminated atmospheres - for escape	Positive-pressure SCBA. Gas mask. Combination positive-pressure SAR with escape SCBA.
Not immediately dangerous to life or health	
Gas and vapor contaminants	Positive-pressure SAR. Gas mask. Chemical-cartridge or canister respirator.
Particulate contaminants	Positive-pressure SAR including abrasive blasting respirator. Powered air-purifying respirator equipped with high-efficiency filters. Any air-purifying respirator with a specific particulate filter.
Gaseous and particulate contaminants	Positive-pressure supplied respirator. Gas mask. Chemical-cartridge respirator with mechanical filters.
Smoke and other fire-related contaminants	Positive-pressure SCBA.

14) Answer B:

The only known health effect associated with exposure to elevated levels of radon is an increased risk of developing lung cancer. The risk of developing lung cancer increases as the level of radon and the length of exposure increase. Radon is not used commercially. Radon is formed by the radioactive decay of certain naturally-occurring uranium and thorium isotopes to radon 222 and eventually to lead 206. Because radon diffuses from the soil and from the domestic water supply, it has become a concern in homes and workplaces. In regions with large deposits of radioactive materials in the ground, radon gas seeps into buildings and decays into radioactive radon daughters.

15) Answer A:
Environmental management guidelines are generally composed of a series of interlinking and supporting components:

- A set of *principles* to help understand environmental management;
- A series of *tools* that can be used to achieve environmental objectives;
- A series of *management programs* traditionally used to solve environmental issues; and
- A *management framework* to integrate environmental issues into the core business processes and decision making

Some tools have been specifically developed as environmental management guidelines (ISO 14001, for example), some have been adopted from other management practices.

16) Answer C:
DOT hazard class 8 is for corrosives and is black and white.

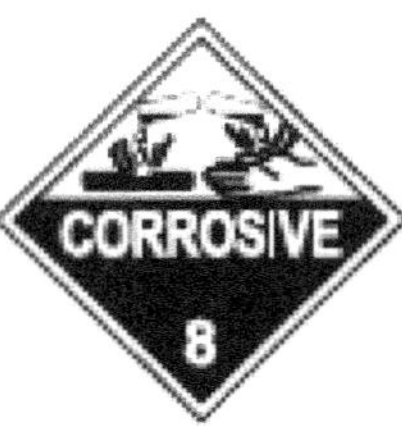

17) Answer A:
According to NIOSH, the best non powered hand tool is one that fits the job you are doing, fits the work space available, and reduces the force you need to apply, fits your hand, and can be used in a comfortable work position.

18) Answer B:
The best solution is to reduce the noise exposure to below the 90 dB exposure based on a time weighted average (TWA). A **noise dosimeter** is used to measure the TWA. When trying to evaluate the impact of high noise levels on the human ear, it is very difficult to determine the effectiveness of hearing protectors. Hearing protectors are evaluated under laboratory conditions specified by ANSI Z24.22 and ANSI S3.19
Using the following formula, evaluate the effectiveness of hearing protection provided to an employee who is using an ear plug assigned a NRR of 37 combined with muffs (NRR = 21) when exposed to an 8 hour TWA of 115 dBA. Note: When two noise reduction devices are used, calculate

attenuation based on the most effective and add 5 for the second. However, in field conditions the ***Noise Reduction Rating (NRR)*** given hearing protectors often is provided a safety factor of 2 or reduced by 50%. This is necessary because field conditions never equal laboratory conditions. Additionally, when two noise reduction devices are properly worn, an additional 5 dB (doubling) of protection is provided. After field attenuation is calculated, it is subtracted from the 8 hour TWA value to obtain the protected TWA (sound level reaching the cochlea). Remember, the exposure limit for baseline is Federal OSHA standard of 90 dBA and 85 dBA if the individual has had a threshold shift. Workers must be properly trained on how to use hearing protection.

$$A_f = \frac{NRR - 7}{2} - 5$$

$$A_f = \frac{37 - 7}{2} - 5$$

$$A_f = 15 - 5$$

$$A_f = 20$$

$$\text{Protected TWA} = TWA_8 - A_f$$

$$\text{Protected TWA} = 115 - 20$$

$$\text{Protected TWA} = 95\ \text{dBA}$$

Under OSHA standards, workers are not permitted to be exposed to an 8-hour TWA equal to or greater than 90 dBA. OSHA uses a 5-dBA exchange rate, meaning the noise level doubles with each additional 5 dBA. The following chart shows how long workers are permitted to be exposed to specific noise levels:

Permissible Duration (Hours per Day)	Sound Level (dBA, Slow Response)
16	85
8	90
4	95
2	100
1.5	102
1	105
0.5	110
0.25 or less	115

19) Answer D:

The following hierarchy of controls are prioritized from most effective to least effective. (**Adapted from ANSI-Z10.2012)**

CONTROLS	EXAMPLES
1. Elimination	Design to eliminate hazards: falls, HAZMAT, confined spaces, materials handling, tools and machinery, etc
2. Substitution	Substitute for less hazardous materials and equipment, reduce energy, etc.
3. Engineering Controls	Incorporate safety trough design such as: Ventilation systems, enclosures, guarding, interlocks, lift tables, conveyors, etc.
4. Warnings	Strategically place signs, alarms, enunciators, labels, etc.
5. Administrative Controls	Standard Operating Procedures (SOPs) such as: Conduct JSAs, job rotation, inspections, training, mentoring, etc.
6. Personal Protective Equipment	PPE assessments may result in the use of: safety glasses, goggles, face shields, fall protection, protective footwear, gloves, respirators, chemical suits, etc.

20) Answer C:

According to NFPA, barricades shall be used in conjunction with safety signs where it is necessary to prevent or limit employee access to work areas containing live parts. Conductive barricades shall not be used where it might cause an electrical hazard. Barricades shall be placed no closer that the Limited Approach. OSHA states that barricades shall be used in conjunction with safety signs where it is necessary to prevent or limit employee access to work areas exposing employees to uninsulated energized conductors or circuit parts. Conductive barricades may not be used where they might cause an electrical contact hazard.

The Flash Protection Boundary (FPB) is the distance at which incident energy is 1.2 cal/cm^2, which is the amount of heat needed to cause second-degree burns. [*NFPA 70E Standard for Electrical Safety in the Workplace. 2012.*]

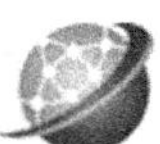

Limited Approach Boundary

Entered only by qualified persons or unqualified persons that have been advised and are escorted by a qualified person. Where one or more unqualified persons are working at or close to the Limited Approach Boundary, the designated person in charge of the workspace where the electrical hazard exists shall cooperate with the designated person in charge of the unqualified person(s) to ensure that all work can be done safely. This shall include advising and warning him or her to stay outside of the Limited Approach Boundary.

Restricted Approach Boundary

Entered only by qualified persons required to use shock protection techniques and PPE

Prohibited Approach Boundary

Entered only by qualified persons requiring same protection as if direct contact with live part

Flash Protection Boundary

Linear distance to prevent any more than 2nd degree burns from a potential arc-flash (typically 4 feet)

Hazard Category	Range of Calculated Incident Energy	Minimum Arc Rating of PPE, cal/cm^2	Clothing Description	Clothing Required
1	>1.2 to 4 cal/cm^2	4 cal/cm^2	Arc - rated clothing, minimum arc rating of 4 cal/cm^2	Fire resistant fabric (FR) Shirt and pants or coveralls
2	>4 to 8 cal/cm^2	8 cal/cm^2	Arc - rated clothing, minimum arc rating of 8 cal/cm ^{2}	Cotton underclothing plus FR shirt and pants
3	>8 to 25 cal/cm^2	25 cal/cm^2	Arc - rated clothing selected so that the system rating meets the required minimum arc rating of 25 cal/cm^2	Cotton underclothing plus FR shirt, pants, coveralls or equivalent
4	>25 to 40 cal/cm^2	40 cal/cm^2	Arc - rated clothing selected so that the system rating meets the required minimum arc rating of 40 cal/cm ^{2}	Cotton underclothing plus FR shirt, pants, plus a multilayer flash suit
Protective Clothing Characteristics based on Source: NFPA 70E. (All details in the NFPA table have not been reproduced.)				

Domain 3 Quiz 4 Questions

1) Compression of nerves and blood vessels between clavicle and first and second ribs is a disease known as:
   A) Polymorphous Light Eruption.
   B) Pneumothorax.
   C) Atelectasis.
   D) Thoracic Outlet Syndrome.

2) A CIH has found that part of the workforce is being exposed to Chromium (VI). Assessment of exposed employees is conducted on Fridays at the shift end. The company CSP should place all test results
   A) On a computer.
   B) In a file cabinet.
   C) In employee's personnel file.
   D) In employee's secured medical record.

3) Which of the following operations requires the **greatest** capture velocity for local exhaust ventilation?
   A) Evaporation from tanks; degreasing; water baths.
   B) Spray booths; intermittent container filling; welding.
   C) Spray painting in shallow booths; barrel filling; crushers.
   D) Grinding; abrasive blasting; tumbling

4) A metal fume hazard potentially present when stainless steel is welded is:
   A) Hexavalent chromium.
   B) Lead chromate.
   C) Zinc oxide.
   D) Magnesium oxide.

5) The **most** dangerous radiation is:
   A) Ionizing.
   B) Non-ionizing.
   C) Electromagnetic.
   D) Radio Frequency.

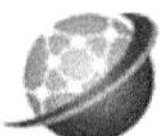

6) Sick building syndrome is defined as:
   A) A lack of sufficient make-up air.
   B) A high level of carbon monoxide.
   C) Formaldehyde that is being released from new carpet at an undesirable rate.
   D) A building in which a significant number of occupants' report illnesses perceived as building related.

7) A waste will be subject to the hazardous waste regulations if it meets any of the following characteristics:
   A) Explosivity, flammability, combustibility, toxicity.
   B) Listed waste, hazardous material, hazardous substance.
   C) Ignitibility, corrosivity, reactivity, or toxicity.
   D) Toxicity, pathogenicity, etiologicity, reactivity.

8) Which is the **best** method to prevent infection from a surface in a lab?
   A) Use of disposable ppe.
   B) Decontamination procedures for ppe.
   C) An industrial hygiene program.
   D) Containment.

9) The **least** common form of cold stress is:
   A) Chilblains caused by temperatures above freezing with high relative humidity that cause itching and redness of the Skin.
   B) Hypothermia caused by below cold temperatures that late lower the body's core temperature.
   C) Frostbite caused extreme cold temperatures that can freeze the skin.
   D) Trench foot caused by cold wet conditions that are above freezing below sixty degrees Fahrenheit.

10) If a person is suffering from heatstroke, which symptom would they **not** experience?
   A) Severe headache.
   B) Profuse sweating and cool moist skin.
   C) Loss of consciousness.
   D) Rapid temperature rise and hot dry skin.

11) The science of measuring the human body for differences in various physical characteristics is:
   A) Kinesiology.
   B) Anthropometry.
   C) Physiology.
   D) Ergonomics.

12) Liver damaging substances such as carbon tetrachloride, chloroform, tannic acid, and trichloroethylene are called?
   A) Nephrotoxins.
   B) Hematoxins.
   C) Hepatotoxins.
   D) Lacrimators.

13) Disorders that affect the muscles, nerves, blood vessels, ligaments and tendons are called:
   A) Chronic wasting disease (CWD).
   B) Musculoskeletal disorders (MSDs).
   C) Cumulative trauma disorders (CTDs).
   D) Soft tissue diseases (STDs).

14) Which of the following groups of hydrocarbons would have the **greatest** chance of not being flammable?
   A) Aliphatic Hydrocarbons.
   B) Aromatic Hydrocarbons.
   C) Halogenated Hydrocarbons.
   D) Ethers.

15) The **best** method for controlling mold in a building is to:
   A) Eliminate the moisture.
   B) Disinfect contaminated materials.
   C) Replace materials that exhibit signs mold growth.
   D) Conduct spore sampling to determine species of mold.

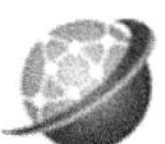

16) LASER is an acronym for:
   A) Luminance Absorption of Stimulated Emitted Radioactivity.
   B) Light Amplification by Stimulated Emission of Radiation.
   C) Light Adsorption by Special Electromagnetic Radiation.
   D) Lumens of Amplified Stimulated Electronic Radioactivity.

17) Insulating rubber gloves must be electrically tested every:
   A) 6 months.
   B) Annual.
   C) Three years.
   D) 90 days.

18) The **most** important consideration when evaluating an emergency practice drill is:
   A) The time of day the drill was conducted.
   B) The number of employees participating in the drill.
   C) The amount of time required to complete the drill.
   D) The communication of the drill by management.

19) Which elements of a task **most** validates the use of PPE as an acceptable control?
   A) Severity of risk and duration of exposure.
   B) Production scheduling.
   C) Budget constraints.
   D) Worker comfort and convenience.

20) Cellular and microwave antennas create non-ionizing radio frequency radiation during transmission that can adversely affect target organs. Which control strategy is **most** effective in eliminating the exposure to workers in the proximity of a powerful radio frequency antenna?
   A) Enforce a two feet approach distance for workers and monitor RF dose.
   B) Limit worker exposure by reducing work duration to less than one hour.
   C) De-energize and lock out the transmitter.
   D) Use lead lined personal protective equipment.

Domain 3 Quiz 4 Answers

1) Answer D:

Thoracic outlet syndrome is defined as a disorder resulting from a compression of nerves and blood vessels between clavicle and first and second ribs at the brachial plexus. It can be caused by typing, keying, carrying heavy loads or keeping the head, arms and/or shoulders in an unnatural position.

2) Answer D:

According to 1910, employee exposure records are part of medical records.
1910.1020(c) (5): "Employee exposure record" means a record containing any of the following kinds of information:
1910.1020(c)(5)(i): Environmental (workplace) monitoring or measuring of a toxic substance or harmful physical agent, including personal, area, grab, wipe, or other form of sampling, as well as related collection and analytical methodologies, calculations, and other background data relevant to interpretation of the results obtained;
1910.1020(c) (5)(ii): Biological monitoring results which directly assess the absorption of a toxic substance or harmful physical agent by body systems (e.g., the level of a chemical in the blood, urine, breath, hair, fingernails, etc.) but not including results which assess the biological effect of a substance or agent or which assess an employee's use of alcohol or drugs;

3) Answer D:

CONDITION OF DISPERSION	EXAMPLES	CAPTURE VELOCITY (FPM)
Released with practically no velocity into quiet air	Evaporation from tanks; degreasing; etc.	50-100
Released at low velocity into moderately still air	Spray booths; intermittent container filling; low speed conveyor transfers; welding; plating; pickling	100-200
Active generation into zone of rapid moving air	Spray painting in shallow booths; barrel filling; conveyor loading; crushers	200-500
Released at high initial velocity into zone of very rapid moving air	Grinding; abrasive blasting; tumbling	500-2000

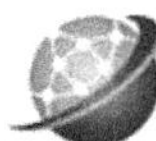

4) Answer A:

According to the NSC *Accident Prevention Manual for* Business *and Industry:* Since chromium is used in all stainless-steel alloys, welding stainless steel can cause fumes of *trivalent or hexavalent form of* chromium to be released into the Welder's breathing zone.

5) Answer A:

Radiation is energy that comes from a source and travels through space at the speed of light. This energy has an electric field and a magnetic field associated with it, and has wave-like properties. You could also call radiation “electromagnetic waves”. Three common measurements of radiation are the amount of radioactivity, ambient radiation levels, and radiation dose. The guiding principle of radiation safety is ALARA or "as low as reasonably achievable".

Roentgen (R)	A measure of energy deposited in tissue/matter Amount of charge from ion particles produced in air Coulombs/Kg air A unit of exposure to ionizing radiation
Radiation Absorbed Dose (RAD)	Amount of absorbed energy deposited in tissue/matter 1 rad = 100 ergs of deposited energy in a gram of tissue/matter 1 gray (Metric) = 100 rads (10,000 ergs) Applicable to all types of radiation
Roentgen Equivalent Man (REM)	Rem is a biologically-weighted absorbed dose. It is a dose equivalent that takes into account the energy absorbed and the biological effect upon tissue. This is especially important in cases of internal exposure. It's often expressed in terms of thousandths of a rem (or mrem). Alpha, beta, and gamma radiation do not all cause the same damage -- they have different biological effects.
As Low As Reasonably Achievable (ALARA)	A principle of safety Limits exposure to radiation as much as possible Ensures that no exposure should be without a benefit

Physiological Effects of radiation include:

- Acute
    - Absorption or intake of a relatively large amount of radiation
    - Over a short amount of time (seconds, minutes, or hours)
- Chronic
    - Absorption or intake of radiation over a long period of time (years or a lifetime)
- Somatic
    - Can occur from acute or chronic exposure
    - Affects the exposed body
    - May be months or years after exposure
    - Shortened life span and aging
    - Can cause cancer
- Genetic
    - May affect future offspring
    - Direct radiation of reproductive organs
    - Cellular DNA affected – mutagenic
- Teratogenic
    - Direct irradiation of developing fetus
    - Results in death or deformity

Whole Body Absorbed Dose (rad)	Effect	Fatalities
10	None	None
100	Nausea, vomiting and diarrhea	None
400	Death without medical intervention	LD50/30
1,000-2,000	Gastrointestinal syndrome	100% in 1 to 2 weeks
Less than 2,000	Central Nervous System	100% in a few days

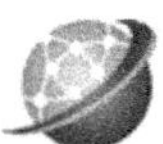

6) Answer D:

Answer D is the American Society of Heating and Air-Conditioning Engineers (ASHRAE) definition of a "Sick Building".
If a significant number of occupants complain of eye, nose, and throat irritation, headaches, dizziness, or difficulty concentrating, but recover soon after leaving the building, these are strong indicators of poor air quality. Buildings with consistently high levels of complaints are commonly called "sick buildings." A Health Hazard Evaluation (HHE) by NIOSH or a similar evaluation by a qualified IAQ test organization will indicate if the building has indoor air quality problems

7) Answer C:

A waste will be subject to the hazardous waste regulations if it meets any of the following conditions: ***Characteristic Waste.*** Waste exhibiting any of the four characteristics of a hazardous waste: ignitibility, corrosivity, reactivity, or toxicity. ***Listed Hazardous Waste.*** Wastes specifically listed in Subpart D of the regulations: Non Specific Source (F-Listed); Specific Source (K-Listed); Acute Hazardous Waste (P-Listed); Toxic Hazardous Waste (U-Listed). ***Mixtures.*** The waste is a mixture of a listed hazardous waste and a non-nonhazardous waste. ***Declared to be Hazardous*. The waste has been declared to be hazardous by the generator.** The Resource Conservation and Recovery Act (RCRA) extended protection to the environmental medium of land. As the name suggests, the law set forth an intent to promote conservation of resources through reduced reliance on landfilling. **This law covers both solid waste and hazardous waste. All hazardous waste is considered solid waste by definition, but not all solid waste is considered hazardous waste.**

8) Answer D:

Containment is the mechanism for ensuring that workers, the immediate work environment, and the community, including those outside the immediate workplace, are protected or shielded from exposure during workplace activities involving infectious or biological agents. As stated in the 5th edition of Biosafety in Microbiological and Biomedical Laboratories (BMBL, 2009), "the term 'containment' is used in describing safe methods, facilities and equipment for managing infectious materials in the laboratory environment where they are being handled or maintained." Varying configurations of these components are used depending on the hazard category of the work. The CDC and NIH have designated four default configurations of work practices, safety equipment, and facility design as biosafety levels (BSLs) for work involving infectious agents or activities in which experimentally or naturally infected vertebrate animals are manipulated. The combination must be specifically appropriate for the operations performed, the documented or suspected routes of transmission of the agent, and the laboratory function or activity. The use of increasingly stringent procedures and more complex laboratory facilities permits higher risk activities to be carried out safely. Specific mitigation measures should be selected based on the identified risks. As a simple example, minimizing sharps would be a good practice for handling an agent that causes disease through percutaneous exposure. Depending on the sophistication of the mitigation measures, containment can be expensive to operate and maintain and/or procedurally burdensome, so optimizing the control measures for the identified risks ideally provide the best return on investment to improve safety.

9) Answer A:

The human body is designed to work optimally at a temperature of 98.6° F ± 1.8°F. The human body is less capable of coping with heart loss than with heat gain. Exposure to cold temperatures, air temperatures less than 61° F, can reduce dexterity manual dexterity. While adaptive mechanisms (i.e. sweating and acclimation) are crucial during heat stress exposures, the physiological adaptations to cold stress have less dramatic effects. The first physiological response to cold stress is to conserve body heat by reducing blood circulation through the skin, effectively making the skin an insulating layer. The second physiological response is boosting the body's metabolism through shivering, a sign of significant cold stress and that hypothermia may be present. However, it is relatively weak as a protective mechanism. Behavior is the primary human response to preventing excessive exposure to cold stress. Behaviors include increasing clothing insulation, increasing activity, and seeking warm locations. Hazards associated with cold stress are manifested in two distinct fashions: systemic (hypothermia) and local (localized tissue damage). As hypothermia progresses, depression of the central nervous system becomes more severe. This accounts for the progression of signs and symptoms from a sluggishness through slurred speech and unsafe behaviors to disorientation and unconsciousness. The ability to sustain metabolic rate and reduced skin blood flow is diminished by fatigue. Thus fatigue increases the risk of severe hypothermia through decreasing metabolic heat and increased heat loss from the skin. Because blood flow through the skin is reduced to conserve heat, the skin and underlying tissues are more susceptible to local cold injury.

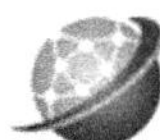

Cold Stress Disorders The four physical disorders that can arise from cold stress, listed in increasing order of severity, are as follows:

- Chilblains: Chilblains usually arise because of inadequate clothing during periods of exposure to cold temperatures and high relative humidity. Reddening of the skin accompanied by localized itching and swelling are the principal indications of chilblains.
- Trench foot, also known as immersion foot, is an injury of the feet resulting from prolonged exposure to wet and cold conditions. Trench foot can occur at temperatures as high as **60 degrees F** if the feet are constantly wet. Injury occurs because wet feet lose heat 25-times faster than dry feet.
- Frostnip: Frostnip, which is like frostbite, results from prolonged, unprotected exposures to cold temperatures above 32°F (0°C). Symptoms of frostnip are areas of pain and/or itching, and a distinct whitening of the skin.
- Frostbite: Frostbite is produced from unprotected exposures to cold temperatures at or below freezing — i.e., ≤32°F or 0°C. Frostbite is characterized by the sequential change in skin color from white to gray to black [depending upon the temperature and the length of exposure], a reduction in the sensations of touch ranging from slight to total [again depending upon the temperature and the length of exposure], and numbness.
- Hypothermia: Hypothermia results from extreme exposures to the factors of cold stress, coupled possibly with dehydration and/or exhaustion. Alcohol and/or drug abuse can also contribute to hypothermia. A person who is experiencing hypothermia will usually show some or all of the following symptoms: chills, euphoria, and pain in the extremities, slow and weak pulse, and body temperature of less than 95°F (35°C), fatigue, drowsiness, and unconsciousness.

Cold-Related Disorders				
Disorder	Symptoms	Signs	Causes	First Aid
Hypothermia	Chills Pain in extremities Fatigue or drowsiness	Euphoria Slow, weak pulse Slurred speech Collapse Shivering Unconsciousness Body temperature <95 F (35 C)	Excessive exposure Exhaustion or dehydration Subnormal tolerance (genetic or acquired) Drug/alcohol abuse	Move to warm area and remove wet clothing Modest external warming (external heat packs, blankets, etc.) Drink warm, sweet fluids if conscious Transport to hospital
Frostbite	Burning sensation at first Coldness, numbness, tingling	Skin color white or grayish yellow to reddish violet to black Blisters Response to touch depends on depth of freezing	Exposure to cold Vascular disease	Move to warm area and remove wet clothing External warming (e.g., warm water Drink warm, sweet fluids if conscious Treat as a burn, do not rub affected area Transport to hospital
Frostnip	Possible itching or pain	Skin turns white	Exposure to cold (above freezing)	Similar to frostbite
Trench Foot	Severe pain Tingling, itching	Edema Blisters Response to touch depends on depth of freezing	Exposure to cold (above freezing) and dampness	Similar to frostbite
Chilblain	Recurrent, localized itching Painful inflammation	Swelling Severe spasms	Inadequate clothing Exposure to cold and dampness Vascular disease	Remove to warm area Consult physician
Raynaud's disorder	Fingers tingle Intermittent blanching and reddening	Fingers blanch with cold exposure	Exposure to cold and vibration Vascular disease	Remove to warm area Consult physician

Hypothermia is related to systemic cold stress, and the other disorders are related to local tissue cooling.

Dressing properly is extremely important to preventing cold stress. The type of fabric worn also makes a difference. Cotton loses its insulation value when it becomes wet. Wool, silk and most synthetics, on the other hand, retain their insulation even when wet.

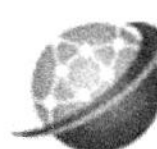

10) Answer B:

Heat Stress Disorders				
Disorder	Symptoms	Signs	Causes	First Aid
Heat stroke	Chills Restlessness Irritability	Euphoria Red face Disorientation Hot, dry skin Erratic behavior Collapse Shivering Unconsciousness Convulsions Body temperature ≥104 F (40 C)	Excessive exposure Subnormal tolerance (genetic or acquired) Drug / alcohol abuse	Immediate, aggressive, effective cooling. Transport to hospital Take body temperature
Heat exhaustion	Fatigue Weakness Blurred vision Dizziness, headache	High pulse rate Profuse sweating Low blood pressure Insecure gait Pale face Collapse Body temperature: Normal to slightly increased	Dehydration (caused by sweating, diarrhea, vomiting) Distribution of blood to the periphery Low level of acclimation Low level of fitness	Lie down flat on back in a cool environment Drink water. Loosen clothing
Dehydration	No early symptoms Fatigue / weakness Dry mouth	Loss of work capacity Increased response time	Excessive fluid loss caused by sweating, illness (vomiting or diarrhea), alcohol consumption	Fluid and salt replacement
Heat syncope	Blurred vision (gray-out) Fainting (brief black-out) Normal temperature	Brief fainting or near-fainting behavior	Pooling of blood in the legs and skin from prolonged static posture and heat exposure	Lie on back in cool environment Drink water
Heat cramps	Painful muscle cramps especially in abdominal or fatigued muscles	Incapacitating pain in muscle	Electrolyte imbalance caused by prolonged sweating without adequate fluid and salt intake	Ret in a cool environment Drink salted water (0.5% salt solution). Massage muscles
Heat rash (prickly heat)	Itching Skin Reduced sweating	Skin eruptions	Prolonged, uninterrupted sweating Inadequate hygiene practices	Keep skin clean and Reduce heat

Heat stress control methods include acclimation, work rest cycles, and rehydration.

11) Answer B:

Anthropometry refers to the measurement of the human individual. Anthropometry involves the systematic measurement of the physical properties of the human body, primarily dimensional descriptors of body size and shape. Today, anthropometry plays an important role in industrial design, clothing design, ergonomics and architecture where statistical data about the distribution of body dimensions in the population are used to optimize products. Changes in lifestyles, nutrition, and ethnic composition of populations lead to changes in the distribution of body dimensions (e.g. the obesity epidemic), and require regular updating of anthropometric data collections.

Kinesiology is a scientific study of human or non-human body movement. Kinesiology addresses physiological, biomechanical, and psychological mechanisms of movement. Applications of kinesiology to human health (i.e. **human Kinesiology**) include biomechanics and orthopedics; strength and conditioning; sport psychology; methods of rehabilitation, such as physical and occupational therapy; and sport and exercise. Studies of human and animal motion include measures from motion tracking systems, electrophysiology of muscle and brain activity, various methods for monitoring physiological function, and other behavioral and cognitive research techniques.

Physiology is the scientific study of the normal function in living systems. A sub-discipline of biology, its focus is in how organisms, organ systems, organs, cells, and biomolecules carry out the chemical or physical functions that exist in a living system

Ergonomics (Human Factors) also known as comfort design, functional design, and systems, is the practice of designing products, systems, or processes to take proper account of the interaction between them and the people who use them. The study of people's efficiency in their working environment. The field has seen contributions from numerous disciplines, such as psychology, engineering, biomechanics, industrial design, physiology, and anthropometry. In essence, it is the study of designing equipment, devices and processes that fit the human body and its cognitive abilities. The two terms "human factors" and "ergonomics" are essentially synonymous.

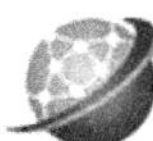

12) Answer C:

Substances capable of damaging the liver are called ***hepatotoxins.*** The liver is the main processing organ for toxins. It may convert toxins into nontoxic forms; however, the liver may generate a more toxic by-product, which can cause cellular and tissue damage. Examples of hepatotoxins are carbon tetrachloride, chloroform, tannic acid, and trichloroethylene. Examples of chemicals that cause cirrhosis (a fibrotic disease that results in liver dysfunction and jaundice) are carbon tetrachloride, alcohol, and aflotoxin. Other effects can range from tumors to enlargement of the liver and fat accumulation. The main function of the kidneys is to filter the blood and eliminate wastes. Because waste gets concentrated in the process, toxins can be at much higher levels in the kidneys. Toxins that damage this organ are known as ***nephrotoxins***. Most heavy metals fall into this category, including mercury, arsenic, and lithium. Many halogenated (i.e., chlorinated) organic compounds are also nephrotoxins such as tetrachloroethylene, carbon tetrachloride, and chloroform. Other chemicals that damage the kidneys include carbon disulfide, methanol, toluene, and ethylene glycol. Substances capable of producing blood disorders are called ***hematoxins***. Chemicals that affect the bone marrow, which is the source of most of the components of blood, are arsenic, bromine, methyl chloride, and benzene. Chemicals that affect platelets, which are cell fragments that help in the process of blood clotting, are aspirin, benzene, and tetrachloroethane. Chemicals that affect white blood cells, which help the body defend against infection, are naphthalene and tetrachloroethane. ***Lacrimators*** are chemicals that can cause instant tearing at low concentrations. Examples are tear gas and MACE. Other chemicals can cause cataracts, optic nerve damage, and retinal damage by circulating through the bloodstream and reaching the eye. Examples of these are naphthalene, methanol, and thallium.

Categories of Hazards in Industrial Toxicology

Class of Hazard	Affected Organ	Possible Signs and Symptoms	Selected Examples
Irritants	Exposed tissues (*e.g.*, mucous tissues)	Pain, fluid accumulation	Acids and acid vapors, sulfur dioxide, ozone, ammonia, chlorine
Simple Asphyxiants	Body cells (O2 is blocked from the lungs)	Confusion, collapse, unconsciousness	Nitrogen, argon, helium, carbon dioxide, methane (natural gas)
Chemical Asphyxiants	Body cells (interferes with oxygenation of body cells)	Confusion, headache, collapse, unconsciousness	Carbon monoxide, hydrogen sulfide, inorganic cyanides
Anesthetics or Central Nervous System Depressants	Central nervous system	Dizziness, drowsiness, collapse, unconsciousness	Liquids and vapors of many organic solvents (*e.g.*, alcohols, ethers, esters, chlorinated hydrocarbons, toluene, xylene, benzene)
Agents that can cause lung illnesses (e.g., fluid accumulation, tissue scarring, cancer)	Lungs, linings of either the lungs or the abdomen	Breathlessness, chest pain, cough, weakness	Asbestos, crystalline silica (*e.g.*, quartz), coal, radioactive substances, beryllium and its compounds, welding fumes, cotton fibers, arsenic and its compounds, hydrogen fluoride, phosgene, nitrogen dioxide
Carcinogens (agents that are known or suspected of causing cancer in humans)	Various organs, depending on the agent	Pain, coughing, tumors, various other symptoms	Confirmed carcinogens include: asbestos, radioactive substances, polycyclic aromatic hydrocarbons (PAHs), arsenic and its compounds, benzene, hexavalent chromium compounds, coal tars and pitches, vinyl chloride Suspect carcinogens include: acrylonitrile, benzidine-based dyes, benzo[a]pyrene, beryllium and its compounds, cadmium and its compounds, carbon tetrachloride, creosote, ethylene oxide, formaldehyde gas, 2,3,7,8- tetrachloro-dibenzo[p]dioxin (TCDD), trichloroethylene, tetrachloroethylene, and crystalline silica dust
Nephrotoxins	Kidneys	Symptoms vary for different agents	Most heavy metals and their compounds (*e.g.*, lead, mercury, chromium, uranium), some halogenated hydrocarbons (*e.g.*,trichloroethylene, chloroform, carbon tetrachloride), 2,4,5-trichlorophenoxyacetic acid (2,4,5-T), polychlorinated biphenyls (PCBs)
Hepatotoxins	Liver	Symptoms vary for different agents	Some halogenated hydrocarbons (*e.g.*, carbon tetrachloride, chloroform, trichloroethylene and tetrachloroethylene), ethyl alcohol, allyl alcohol, urethane monomer, hydrazine, cerium and its compounds, beryllium and its compounds, and some pharmaceuticals
Chemical Allergens (sensitizers)	Various tissues, especially skin and eyes	Itching, swelling, inflammation	Formaldehyde, beryllium and its compounds, toluene-2,4-diisocyanate (TDI), creosote, some acrylates, epoxy resins and components, coal tar and its derivatives, some organic dyes, turpentine, some woods, poison ivy and oak, white sumac, some pharmaceuticals
Genotoxic and fetotoxic agents	Genotoxic: affects the genetic material of reproductive cells Fetotoxic: affects a fetus	Genotoxins: may be few immediate signs Fetotoxins: deformity or loss of a fetus	Benzene, toluene, xylene, ethyl alcohol, carbon disulfide, carbon monoxide, lead and its compounds, mercury and its compounds, arsenic and its compounds, cadmium and its compounds, radiation and radioactive substances, chlorinated phenoxyacetic acids, paraquat, diquat, PCBs, TCDD, ethylene oxide, dinitrobenzene, and some pharmaceuticals

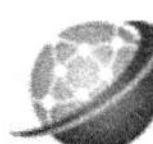

13) Answer B:

Examples of Musculoskeletal Disorders				
Body Parts Affected	Symptoms	Possible Causes	Workers Affected	Disease Name
thumbs	pain at the base of the thumbs	twisting and gripping	butchers, housekeepers, packers, seamstresses, cutters	De Quervain's disease
fingers	difficulty moving finger; snapping and jerking movements	repeatedly using the index fingers	meatpackers, poultry workers, carpenters, electronic assemblers	trigger finger
shoulders	pain, stiffness	working with the hands above the head	power press operators, welders, painters, assembly line workers	rotator cuff tendinitis
hands, wrists	pain, swelling	repetitive or forceful hand and wrist motions	core making, poultry processing, meatpacking	tenosynovitis
fingers, hands	numbness, tingling; ashen skin; loss of feeling and control	exposure to vibration	chain saw, pneumatic hammer, and gasoline powered tool operators	Raynaud's syndrome (white finger)
fingers, wrists	tingling, numbness, severe pain; loss of strength, sensation in the thumbs, index, or middle or half of the ring fingers	repetitive and forceful manual tasks without time to recover	meat and poultry and garment workers, upholsterers, assemblers, VDT operators, cashiers	carpal tunnel syndrome
back	low back pain, shooting pain or numbness in the upper legs	whole body vibration	truck and bus drivers, tractor and subway operators; warehouse workers; nurses' aides; grocery cashiers; baggage handlers	back disability

Musculoskeletal disorders (MSDs) affect the muscles, nerves, blood vessels, ligaments and tendons. Workers in many different industries and occupations can be exposed to risk factors at work, such as lifting heavy items, bending, reaching overhead, pushing and pulling heavy loads, working in awkward body postures and performing the same or similar tasks repetitively. Exposure to these known risk factors for MSDs increases a worker's risk of injury. MSDs are very difficult to define within traditional disease classifications. These disorders have received many names, such as:

- Repetitive motion injuries.
- Repetitive strain injuries.
- Cumulative trauma disorders.
- Occupational cervicobrachial disorders.
- Overuse syndrome.
- Regional musculoskeletal disorders.
- Soft tissue disorders.

Most of the names do not accurately describe the disorders. For example, the term "repetitive strain injuries" suggests that repetition causes these disorders, but awkward postures also contribute. These terms are used synonymously, however, MSD term is used in current literature. Work-related MSDs can be prevented. Ergonomics, fitting a job to a person, helps lessen muscle fatigue, increases productivity and reduces the number and severity of work-related MSDs.

Bureau of Labor Statistics (BLS) defines musculoskeletal disorders (MSDs) to include cases where the nature of the injury or illness is pinched nerve; herniated disc; meniscus tear; sprains, strains, tears; hernia (traumatic and nontraumatic); pain, swelling, and numbness; carpal or tarsal tunnel syndrome; Raynaud's syndrome or phenomenon; musculoskeletal system and connective tissue diseases and disorders, when the event or exposure leading to the injury or illness is overexertion and bodily reaction, unspecified; overexertion involving outside sources; repetitive motion involving microtasks; other and multiple exertions or bodily reactions; and rubbed, abraded, or jarred by vibration.

The risk of MSD injury depends on work positions and postures, how often the task is performed, the level of required effort and how long the task lasts. Risk factors that may lead to the development of MSDs include:

- **Exerting excessive force**. Examples include lifting heavy objects or people, pushing or pulling heavy loads, manually pouring materials, or maintaining control of equipment or tools.
- **Performing the same or similar tasks repetitively**. Performing the same motion or series of motions continually or frequently for an extended period of time.
- **Working in awkward postures or being in the same posture for long periods of time**. Using positions that place stress on the body, such as prolonged or repetitive reaching above shoulder height, kneeling, squatting, and leaning over a counter, using a knife with wrists bent, or twisting the torso while lifting.

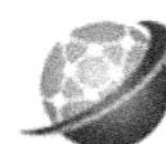

- **Localized pressure into the body part**. Pressing the body or part of the body (such as the hand) against hard or sharp edges, or using the hand as a hammer.
- **Cold temperatures**. In combination with any one of the above risk factors may also increase the potential for MSDs to develop. For example, many of the operations in meatpacking and poultry processing occur with a chilled product or in a cold environment.
- **Vibration**. Both whole body and hand-arm, can cause a number of health effects. Hand-arm vibration can damage small capillaries that supply nutrients and can make hand tools more difficult to control. Hand-arm vibration may cause a worker to lose feeling in the hands and arms resulting in increased force exertion to control hand-powered tools (e.g. hammer drills, portable grinders, chainsaws) in much the same way gloves limit feeling in the hands. The effects of vibration can damage the body and greatly increase the force which must be exerted for a task.
- **Combined exposure to several risk factors**. May place workers at a higher risk for MSDs than does exposure to any one risk factor.

To reduce the chance of injury, work tasks should be designed to limit exposure to ergonomic risk factors. Engineering controls are the most desirable, where possible. Administrative or work practice controls may be appropriate in some cases where engineering controls cannot be implemented or when different procedures are needed after implementation of the new engineering controls. Personal protection solutions have only limited effectiveness when dealing with ergonomic hazards.

Chronic wasting disease (**CWD**) is a transmissible spongiform encephalopathy (TSE) of mule deer, white-tailed deer, elk, and moose. As of 2016, CWD had only been found in members of the deer family. CWD is typified by chronic weight loss leading to death. No relationship is known between CWD and any other TSE of animals or people. Although reports in the popular press have been made of humans being affected by CWD, a study by the Centers for Disease Control and Prevention suggests, "[m]ore epidemiologic and laboratory studies are needed to monitor the possibility of such transmissions." The epidemiological study further concluded, "[a]s a precaution, hunters should avoid eating deer and elk tissues known to harbor the CWD agent (e.g., brain, spinal cord, eyes, spleen, tonsils, lymph nodes) from areas where CWD has been identified.

14) Answer C:

Hydrocarbons are compounds that contain atoms of carbon and hydrogen only. They are broadly classified into two types, that is; aliphatic and aromatic. *Aliphatic hydrocarbons* are subdivided into saturated and unsaturated compounds and include the alkanes: methane, ethane, propane and butane. ***Aromatic hydrocarbons*** are derivative of the parent compound benzene. ***Ethers*** are members of a class of organic compound in which an oxygen atom has bridged between two hydrocarbon groups. Aliphatic ethers are highly volatile and extremely flammable. Hydrocarbons that have been partially halogenated burn, but generally with much less ease than their nonhalogenated analogs. The fully ***halogenated*** derivatives such as carbon tetrachloride are non-combustible.

15) Answer A:

Molds can live for years in a dormant state. To grow, the spores need moisture, warm temperature, low air movement, and a food source. Eliminating moisture is the best method of control. Molds can become airborne when their habitats are disturbed by shaking or sweeping. The airborne molds can travel with air current, land on surfaces, and settle into the tiniest cracks and crevices of carpets, furniture, draperies, insulation, rough textures, and smooth surfaces. Heating and cooling ducts, wet carpets, damp upholstery, and air filters on air conditioners and furnaces become common habituating places for molds. Exposure to mold spores may cause allergy (hypersensitivity reaction), poisoning (if the spores contain mycotoxins), or infection. Some spores infect healthy hosts; others infect mostly compromised hosts. A combination of these responses is possible. Many airborne molds in indoor environments are responsible for human respiratory allergies. Reactions to molds can result in sneezing, itching, coughing, wheezing, shortness of breath, and chest pain. Molds are measured in spores/m^3.

16) Answer B:

LASER is an acronym which stands for Light Amplification by Stimulated Emission of Radiation. The laser produces an intense, highly directional beam of light. The most common cause of laser-induced tissue damage is thermal in nature, where the tissue proteins are denatured due to the temperature rise following absorption of laser energy. Laser work and similar operations create intense concentrations of heat, ultraviolet, infrared, and reflected light radiation. A laser beam, of sufficient power, can produce intensities greater than those experienced when looking directly at the sun. Unprotected laser exposure may

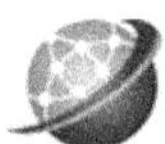

result in eye injuries including retinal burns, cataracts, and permanent blindness. ANSI Z136.1 (Safe Use of Lasers) Laser eyewear must be selected with the specific laser wave length in mind. The International Electro-technical Commission (IEC) publishes standards on laser safety. The IEC also sets out five classes of laser: 1, 2, 3A, 3B and 4. This classification gives the user an indication of the degree of laser hazard.

- **Class 1** lasers have an output power that is below the level at which eye injury can occur.
- **Class 2** lasers emit visible light and are limited to a maximum output power of 1-milliwatt (mW). A person receiving an eye exposure from a Class 2 laser will be protected from injury by their natural blink reflex, an involuntary response which causes the person to blink and turn their head, thereby avoiding eye exposure.
- **Class 3A** lasers may have a maximum output power of 5 mW. This limit restricts the power entering a fully dilated human eye (taken as a 7 mm aperture) to 1 mW. Thus, accidental exposure to a Class 3A laser should be no more hazardous than exposure to a Class 2 laser. However, Class 3A laser pointers are hazardous when viewed with an optical aid such as binoculars and are therefore unsuitable for the general consumer.
- **Class 3B** lasers have an **output power up to 500 mW, sufficient to cause eye injury.** The extent and severity of any eye injury will depend upon several factors including the laser power entering the eye and the exposure duration.
    - Class 1, Class 2, Class 3A and Class 3B lasers do not have sufficient power to cause a skin injury.
- **Class 4** lasers have an output power greater than 500 mW are capable of causing injury to both the eye and skin and will be a fire hazard if sufficiently high output powers are available.

17) Answer A:

Testing and Inspection. Gloves and sleeves must be electrically tested before being issued for use. They must also be visually inspected and gloves need to be air tested for any possible defects (for example, cuts, holes, tears, embedded objects, changes in texture) before each day's use and whenever there is a reason to believe they may have been damaged. Best practice is to inspect PPE and air test the gloves and sleeves before each use. [See 1910.137(b)(2)].

- Insulating equipment may not be used if any of the following defects are present: holes, tears, punctures or cuts, ozone cutting or ozone checking, embedded foreign objects, texture changes, including swelling, softening, hardening, or becoming sticky or inelastic, and any other defect that damages the insulating properties. [See 1910.137(b)(2)(iii) and ASTM

F1236-96, Standard Guide for Visual Inspection of Electrical Protective Rubber Products].

- Insulating equipment failing to pass inspection must be removed from service and may not be used by workers.

In addition, the gloves and sleeves must be electrically tested at regular intervals of not more than 6 months for gloves and 12 months for sleeves. (See ASTM F496, Standard Specification for In-Service Care of Insulating Gloves and Sleeves for some appropriate test methods.) When gloves and sleeves are used regularly, best practice is to test as frequently as monthly. [See 1910.137(b)(2)]

18) Answer C:

Emergencies can create a variety of hazards for workers in the impacted area. Preparing before an emergency incident plays a vital role in ensuring that employers and workers have the necessary equipment, know where to go, and know how to keep themselves safe when an emergency occurs. Before implementing the emergency plans, the employer must designate and train enough people to assist in the safe and orderly emergency evacuation of employees. Employers should review the plan with each employee when the initial plan is developed and when each employee is initially assigned to the job. Employers should review the plan with each employee when his/her actions or responsibilities under the plan change or when the plan changes. Effective plans often call for retraining employees annually and include drills in which employees can practice evacuating their workplace and gathering in the assembly area. Be sure all employees understand the function and elements of your emergency action plan, including types of potential emergencies, reporting procedures, alarm systems, evacuation plans, and shutdown procedures. Discuss any special hazards you may have onsite such as flammable materials, toxic chemicals, radioactive sources, or water-reactive substances. Clearly communicate to your employees who will be in charge during an emergency to minimize confusion.

- General training for your employees should also address the following:
- Individual roles and responsibilities.
- Threats, hazards, and protective actions.
- Notification, warning, and communications procedures.
- Means for locating family members in an emergency.
- Emergency response procedures.
- Evacuation, shelter, and accountability procedures.

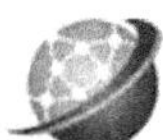

- Location and use of common emergency equipment.
- Emergency shutdown procedures.

Once you have reviewed your emergency action plan with your employees and everyone has had the proper training, it is a good idea to hold practice drills as often as necessary to keep employees prepared. Include outside resources such as fire and police departments when possible. After each drill, gather management and employees to evaluate the effectiveness of the drill. Identify the strengths and weaknesses of your plan and work to improve it. The most important concepts of emergency evacuation include:

- Establish assembly points and equipment (such as fire extinguishers, first aid kits, and spill kits) that may be needed in an emergency. Most employers create maps from floor diagrams with arrows that designate the exit route assignments.
- Exit routes should be clearly marked and well lit, wide enough to accommodate the number of evacuating personnel, unobstructed and clear of debris at all times, and unlikely to expose evacuating personnel to additional hazards.
- Accounting for all employees following an evacuation is critical. Confusion in the assembly areas can lead to delays in rescuing anyone trapped in the building, or unnecessary and dangerous search-and-rescue operations. To ensure the fastest, most accurate accounting of your employees, consider taking a head count after the evacuation.

(How to Plan for Workplace Emergencies and Evacuations OSHA Publication 3088)

19) Answer A:

PPE includes a variety of devices and garments to protect workers from injuries. PPE is designed to protect eyes, face, head, ears, feet, hands and arms, and the whole body. PPE includes such items as goggles, face shields, safety glasses, hard hats, safety shoes, gloves, vests, earplugs, earmuffs, and suits for full-body protection. Hazard analysis and assessment procedures shall be used to assess the workplace to determine if hazards are present, or are likely to be present, which may necessitate the use of PPE. As part of this assessment, employees' work environment is to be examined for potential hazards, both health and physical, the severity of hazards and duration of exposure. If it is not possible to eliminate workers' exposure or potential exposure to the hazard through the efforts of engineering controls, work practices, and administrative controls, then proper PPE will need to be selected, issued, and worn. For example after all feasible engineering controls are implements, such as noise enclosures, than hearing protection is commonly be used to attenuate the noise to below the exposure limit. The use of PPE should be the last consideration in eliminating or reducing the hazards the employee is subjected to because PPE can be heavy, awkward, uncomfortable, and expensive to maintain. (Reese, 2003)

20) Answer C:
To minimize the risk of adverse health effects, radiofrequency (RF) fields as well as induced and contact currents must be in compliance with applicable guidelines (e.g., ICNIRP, ANSI, ACGIH). Reduction in RF exposures can be accomplished through the implementation of appropriate, administrative, work practice and engineering controls. These various controls are the elements of an RF Protection Program, and part of an employer's comprehensive safety and health program. According to OSHA, EPA and various consensus standards, control of RF hazards include:

- Controlling exposure time and the distance between the RF source and the operator are important in maintaining workers' exposures below recommended levels. When necessary due to excessive leakage, "RF hazard areas" must be identified to alert workers of areas that are not to be occupied during RF application. The location of the hazard areas must be based on exposure measurements made during maximum field generation and duty factor (i.e., ratio of RF "on" time during any 6 minute period, assuming intermittent exposure).
- Access to RF hazard areas should be controlled with standard Lockout/Tagout procedures (ref. 29 CFR 1910.147) to ensure workers are not occupying these areas during the application of RF energy. It may be possible to use continuous monitors and/or personal monitors in lieu of, or to supplement, more traditional Lockout/Tagout procedures which lockout the RF power source.
- The RF hazard areas shall be clearly marked with appropriate signs, barricades, floor markings, etc. such that any worker who has access to the facility will be alerted not to occupy the hazardous locations. Signs shall be of standard design and shape (ref ANSI C95. 1), and of sufficient size to be recognizable and readable from a safe distance.
- Screening measurements can be used to determine where to locate signs to alert workers approaching an RF hazard area, including the appropriate warning message on the sign (e.g., Notice, Caution, and Danger).
- The evacuation of hazard areas prior to RF application must be strictly enforced. For example, a procedure which requires an RF sealer operator to

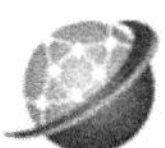

first load the sealer, step back 2 meters to get outside the RF hazard area prior to activating the RF energy, and then walk back to unload the sealer will be difficult to enforce.

Radiofrequency (RF) and microwave (MW) radiation are electromagnetic radiation in the frequency ranges 3 kilohertz (kHz) - 300 Megahertz (MHz), and 300 MHz - 300 gigahertz (GHz), respectively. Research continues on possible biological effects of exposure to RF/MW radiation from radios, cellular phones, the processing and cooking of foods, heat sealers, vinyl welders, and high frequency welders, induction heaters, flow solder machines, communications transmitters, radar transmitters, ion implant equipment, microwave drying equipment, sputtering equipment and glue curing. There are no specific OSHA standards for radiofrequency and microwave radiation issues.

The American National Standards Institute (ANSI) publishes consensus standards on radiofrequency (RF) exposures and measurements. The Institute of Electrical and Electronics Engineers (IEEE) is the co-secretariat for ANSI for developing radiofrequency (RF) standards. ANSI C95.6-2002, Safety Levels with Respect to Human Exposure to Electromagnetic Fields, 0-3 kHz, defines exposure levels to protect against adverse effects in humans from exposure to electric and magnetic fields at frequencies from 0 to 3 kHz. The basis for current RF OSHA standards is based on animal behavioral disruption threshold. It is based on the power that raises body temperature no more than 1° C. With a 10-fold safety factor, it is calculated by 0.4 W/Kg whole body weight. Localized max is 20 times the whole body average or 8 W/Kg. At 3 – 6 GHz frequency, the body becomes a good antenna, which maximizes absorption. Radiation protection guidance is given in 29 CFR 1910.97. Under normal environmental conditions and for incident electromagnetic energy of frequencies from 10 MHz to 100 GHz, the radiation protection guide is 10 mW/cm^2 (milliwatt per square centimeter) as averaged over any possible 0.1-hour period. This guide applies whether the radiation is continuous or intermittent. The guide also mandates the appearance of RF signs to be posted (ANSI C95.2). These formulated recommendations pertain to both whole body irradiation and partial body irradiation, meaning measurable exposure. Partial body irradiation must be included because it has been shown that some parts of the human body (e.g., eyes, testicles) may be harmed if exposed to incident radiation levels significantly in excess of the recommended levels. (Snyder, 2013)

Domain 4: Incident Investigation and Emergency Preparedness

Domain 4: Incident Investigation and Emergency Preparedness 11.5%
Knowledge of: 1. Fundamentals of causal analysis (e.g., 5 whys, root cause analysis) 2. Components or elements of an effective incident/accident management program 3. Emergency action requirements/procedures (e.g., response plans, evacuations, preparedness, operation upsets) 4. Components or elements of an emergency response plan (e.g., roles and responsibilities, emergency contact information, stakeholder notification, media response) 5. Incident command structure in emergency response 6. Techniques for identifying gaps in an emergency response plan (e.g., table top drills, lessons learned) 7. Basic elements of workers' compensation and case management programs
Skill to: 1. Calculate incident and injury rates

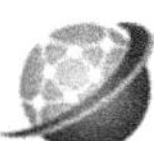

Incident Investigation

Incident is a term used to describe any unplanned event that either results in personal injury or damage to property, equipment, or the environment, or has the *potential* to result in such consequences. Root cause analysis that uses experience, logic, and reasoning to determine which conditions or events, if controlled, will prevent the recurrence of an incident.

A basic 5 step approach to incident investigation includes:

1). Respond safely to the incident
- Assess the scene
- Care for the injured
- Responder safety
- Secure the area
- Preserve the evidence

2). Investigate the incident
- Review camera footage
- Interview Witnesses
- Review operational data
- Documentation

3). Analyze the data and determine root causes
- Multiple causation: People; Equipment: Environment; Management System Errors
- Recommend corrective action
- Identify enhancers and barriers to corrective actions

4). Implement recommendations
- Prevention through hierarchy of controls
- Get shareholder buy in
- Communicate the recommendations
- Standardize the changes

5). Follow up
- Verify controls are implemented
- Discussions with share holders
- Observations

Emergency Preparedness

Hazard prevention and control includes planning to protect employees during foreseeable emergencies, such as fires and explosions, chemical releases, hazardous material spills, unplanned equipment shutdowns, natural disasters, weather emergencies, and medical emergencies.

Some workplaces may already have formal written emergency response plans, as required by authorities such as local fire and emergency response departments, state agencies, the U.S.
Environmental Protection Agency, and OSHA establish requirements for Emergency Action Plans, Fire Prevention Plans, and Emergency Response Plans to ensure that emergency responders and employees know what to do in an emergency.

Regular drills are needed to train employees in proper procedures during emergencies. Drills also provide a way to test the emergency plan and make sure that it is effective at mitigating hazards and moving employees out of potential danger zones. After each drill and following any actual emergency, the plan's effectiveness should be reviewed. Any needed changes, revisions, and updates to the plan should be made in response to these reviews or to changing circumstances within the workplace.

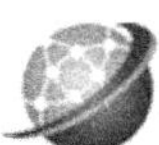

Domain 4 Quiz 1 Questions

1) A company has experienced 90 cases involving days away, restricted or transferred after working a total of 1,623,451 hours. Based on 200,000 hours, calculate is the DART incident rate.
   A) 11.1
   B) 21.8
   C) 17.4
   D) 9.01

2) A company has worked 305,000 hours and has experienced 8 lost work day cases. Based on 1,000,000 hours worked, what is the severity rate for lost workday cases?
   A) 5.25
   B) 10.50
   C) 34.46
   D) 26.23

3) What type of extinguisher is used for an incipient stage aluminum powder fire?
   A) Class C.
   B) Class D.
   C) Class K.
   D) Class B.

4) The smaller the particle size of combustible dust in a confined space:
   A) Has no impact on the explosion hazard.
   B) Has an impact on the explosion only if settled in the space.
   C) Has a lesser impact for a weaker explosion.
   D) Has a greater impact for more a powerful explosion.

5) The **best** fire protection policy for building construction, alteration, or demolition is/are provided by:
   A) Sprinklers that are operational in as many building areas as possible.
   B) Fire bottles available on all floors.
   C) The Fire Marshal making monthly visits to all construction or demolition areas.
   D) A fire watch hired as soon as debris starts to accumulate.

6) The characterization of a Class II, Division 2 location, according to the National Electrical Code is?
   A) A site where flammable or combustible vapors may be present in sufficient quantities to be hazardous.
   B) A place where combustible dust is normally present in adequate quantities to be hazardous.
   C) A scene where flammable or combustible vapors are not normally present, but could be, due to atypical or intermittent operations.
   D) A location where combustible dust is not normally present but with the potential due to abnormal or periodic operations.

7) The fire tetrahedron states that combustion requires an oxidizer, fuel, heat and:
   A) Confinement.
   B) Surface area.
   C) Chain reaction.
   D) Deflagration.

8) A rate-of-rise detector responds to which condition?
   A) Smoke particulate in the air.
   B) Water pressure in fire suppression piping.
   C) Indoor humidity.
   D) Heat.

9) Four components must be present for a chemical explosion to occur. These are an oxidizer, fuel, ignition source and
   A) Overpressure.
   B) Confinement.
   C) Reduction.
   D) Detonation

10) Which types of questions are **most** important for an interviewer to use during an incident investigation?
   A) Reflective.
   B) Open ended.
   C) Guided.
   D) Close ended.

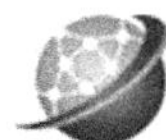

11) Immediately following an incident investigation, the investigator prints the digital pictures taken at the scene and makes notes on the pictures describing the context, orientation of the photographer, lighting, date, time and other information that may be helpful later in the investigation. What does this process describe?
   A) Chain of custody procedures.
   B) Spoiled evidence protocols.
   C) Forensic quality procedures.
   D) Evidentiary preservation regulations.

12) All of the following are valid reasons for accident (mishap) investigation **except**?
   A) Prevent reoccurrence of similar events.
   B) Establish causal factors.
   C) Provide vehicle for discipline.
   D) Provide data for trend analysis.

13) A new operations safety manager has been asked to develop an incident data collection system. The essential **first** step in this process is:
   A) Identify existing data sources and codify the data.
   B) Establish incident reporting procedures.
   C) Define the subsequent use of the data.
   D) Define investigation team parameters.

14) A manufacturing operation is experiencing above average incident and accident occurrences at specific location. The **first** step for implementation of actions to reduce these occurrences is to?
   A) Survey the facility to determine the probable cause of the injuries.
   B) Bring a safety committee on-line to handle the problems.
   C) Train all line supervisors in accident/incident prevention.
   D) Schedule a meeting with upper management to discuss the situation.

15) The Critical Incident Technique method employed during an incident investigation is:
   A) A technique to identify mechanical reliability issues in chemical process machinery.
   B) An open-ended retrospective method of interviews that identify the critical aspects of an incident.
   C) A prescribed dialogue as part of pre-emergency planning exercises.
   D) A sampling of individual behaviors through observations.

16) A characteristic of a root cause for an event or incident is:
   A) Human error.
   B) A management system problem.
   C) An error made by a manager or supervisor.
   D) Intentional unsafe act performed by an employee or work team.

17) In the history of chemical and petroleum industries, causal factors for major events have often related to inadequacies in these four management processes:
   A) Maintenance of mechanical integrity; action items follow-up; management of change; process safety training and competency.
   B) Near miss reports, accident trends analysis, incident investigation reports, management of change.
   C) Training assessment, near miss reports, leading indicators, lagging indicators.
   D) Leading indicators, accident reports, balanced score cards, behavior based observations.

18) When calculating the total case incident rate, the numerator of the formula is:
   A) The number of lost workdays multiplied by 100 employees working 200 hours per year.
   B) The number of cases involving days away from work, transfer, and work restriction multiplied by 200,000.
   C) The actual hours worked multiplied by the total number of cases.
   D) The number of cases multiplied by 100 employees working 2000 hours per year.

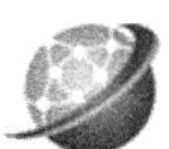

19) The 5-Whys is an iterative question-asking technique used to explore the cause-and-effect relationships underlying a particular problem used to identify which of the following?
    A) Root causes of incidents.
    B) Outcomes of incidents.
    C) Behavior-based safety rules.
    D) Human behavior errors.

20) When it is not possible to interview people at the accident site, what is the next **best** place to interview a witness?
    A) Break room.
    B) Conference room.
    C) Your office.
    D) Supervisor's office.

Domain 4 Quiz 1 Answers

1) Answer A:

$$\text{Rate} = \frac{\text{Cases} \times 200{,}000}{\text{Total hours worked}}$$

$$\text{Rate} = \frac{90 \times 200{,}000}{1{,}623{,}451}$$

$$\text{Rate} = \frac{18{,}000{,}000}{1{,}623{,}451}$$

$$\text{Rate} = 11.1$$

The incidence rate for lost workday cases is the most meaningful lagging performance indicator for a safety program. Days away restricted or transferred cases are an indicator of severity of the injury.

2) Answer D:
Apply formula and compute severity rate.
(8 x 1,000,000)/305,000 = 26.23

$$\text{Rate} = \frac{\text{LWD cases} \times 1{,}000{,}000}{\text{Total hours worked}}$$

$$\text{Rate} = \frac{8 \times 1{,}000{,}000}{305{,}000}$$

$$\text{Rate} = \frac{8{,}000{,}000}{305}$$

$$\text{Rate} = 26.23$$

This means that the business severity rate is 26.23 LWD cases for every 1,000,000 hours worked per year.

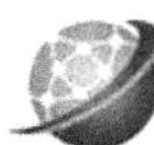

3) Answer B:

Aluminum powders have the highest K_{ST} rate (a measurement of inherent explosive power) of all the combustible metal dusts. The designation "dry powder" has been especially chosen to indicate an agent's suitability for use on Class D (combustible metal) fires. The term "dry chemical" is reserved for agents effective on A:B:C or B:C fires.

FIRE TYPE	EXTINGUISHING AGENT	EXTINGUISHING METHOD
ORDINARY SOLID MATERIALS A	WATER FOAM	REMOVES HEAT REMOVES AIR AND HEAT
	DRY CHEMICAL	BREAKS CHAIN REACTION
FLAMMABLE LIQUIDS B	FOAM CO_2	REMOVES AIR
	DRY CHEMICAL HALON	BREAKS CHAIN REACTION
ELECTRICAL EQUIPMENT C	CO_2	REMOVES AIR
	DRY CHEMICAL HALON	BREAKS CHAIN REACTION
COMBUSTIBLE METALS D	SPECIAL AGENTS	USUALLY REMOVE AIR

4) Answer D:

Combustible dust is defined as a solid material composed of distinct particles or pieces, regardless of size, shape, or chemical composition, which presents a fire or deflagration hazard when suspended in air or some other oxidizing medium over a range of concentrations. Combustible dusts are often either organic or metal dusts that are finely ground into very small particles, fibers, fines, chips, chunks, flakes, or a small mixture of these. As discussed in OSHA's Safety and Health Information Bulletin (SHIB): *Combustible Dust in Industry: Preventing and Mitigating the Effects of Fire and Explosions*, dust particles with an effective diameter of less than 420 microns (those passing through a U.S. No. 40 standard sieve) should be deemed to meet the criterion of the definition. However, larger particles can still pose a deflagration hazard (for instance, as larger particles are moved, they can abrade each other, creating smaller particles). In addition, particles can stick together (agglomerate) due to electrostatic charges accumulated through handling, causing them to become explosible when dispersed. Types of dusts include, but are not limited to: metal dust, such as aluminum and magnesium; wood dust; plastic or rubber dust; biosolids; coal dust; organic dust, such as flour, sugar, paper, soap, and dried blood; and dusts from certain textiles. Five elements are necessary to initiate a dust explosion, often referred to as the "Dust Explosion Pentagon".

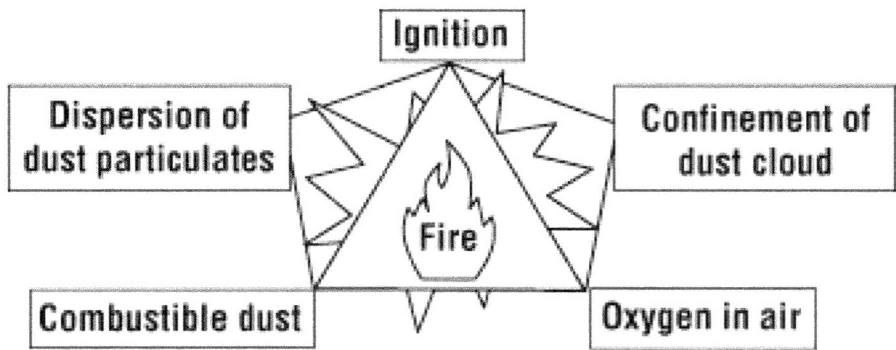

The first three elements are those needed for a fire

1. Combustible dust (fuel);
2. Ignition source (heat); and,
3. Oxygen in air (oxidizer).

An additional two elements must be present for a combustible dust explosion:

4. Dispersion of dust particles in sufficient quantity and concentration; and,
5. Confinement of the dust cloud.

If one of the above five elements is missing, an explosion cannot occur. The ease of ignition and the severity of a combustible dust explosion are typically influenced by particle size. Other factors that influence the explosiveness of dusts include moisture content, ambient humidity, oxygen available for combustion, the shape of dust particles, and the concentration of dust in the air. The actual class is sample specific and will depend on varying characteristics of the material such as particle size or moisture.

* OSHA CPL 03-00-008 - Combustible Dust National Emphasis Program.

** NFPA 68, Standard on Explosion Prevention by Deflagration Venting.

Specific guidance measures to prevent explosions can be found in OSHA's SHIB *Combustible Dust in Industry: Preventing and Mitigating the Effects of Fire and Explosions*, which lists measures to control dusts, eliminate ignition sources, and limit the effects of explosions to minimize injuries. Initial preventative steps are to contain combustible dust to areas that are properly designed and located, with ignition sources either eliminated or controlled. Equipment or spaces such as ducts, dust collectors, vessels, and processing equipment that contain combustible dust should be designed in a manner to prevent leaks to minimize the escape of dust into work areas. Any dust that settles on workplace surfaces should be removed through a routinely

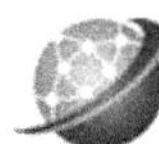

implemented housekeeping program. Areas or equipment potentially subject to explosions, including the dust collection system, should also be designed to relieve pressure in a safe manner, or be provided with proper suppression, explosion prevention systems, or an oxygen-deficient atmosphere. The current definition in NFPA 654 is "a combustible particulate solid that presents a fire or deflagration hazard when suspended in air or some other oxidizing medium over a range of concentrations, regardless of particle size or shape." The same definition is used for combustible metal dust in NFPA 484, *Standard for Combustible Metals, Metal Powders, and Metal Dusts* contains comprehensive guidance on the control of dusts to prevent explosions. The following are some of its recommendations:

- Minimize the escape of dust from process equipment or ventilation systems;
- Use dust collection systems and filters;
- Utilize surfaces that minimize dust accumulation and facilitate cleaning;
- Provide access to all hidden areas to permit inspection;
- Inspect for dust residues in open and hidden areas, at regular intervals;
- Clean dust residues at regular intervals;
- Use cleaning methods that do not generate dust clouds, if ignition sources are present;
- Only use vacuum cleaners approved for dust collection;
- Locate relief valves away from dust hazard areas; and
- Develop and implement a hazardous dust inspection, testing, housekeeping, and control program (preferably in writing with established frequency and methods).

Facilities should carefully identify the following in order to assess their potential for dust explosions:

- Materials that can be combustible when finely divided;
- Processes which use, consume, or produce combustible dusts;
- Open areas where combustible dusts may build up;
- Hidden areas where combustible dusts may accumulate;
- Means by which dust may be dispersed in the air; and
- Potential ignition sources.

5) Answer A:

The threat of fire during construction, alteration or demolition projects is extremely high due to the presence of large quantities of combustible materials and debris and the many ignition sources available from construction or destruction operations. Additionally, the arson threat is greater during construction than at any other time. The maintenance of an operational fire sprinkler system with adequate water supply is the single most important fire prevention action one can take during these operations. Fire sprinklers should be the first system enabled and the last system disabled during construction or demolition.

6) Answer D:
Class II, Division 2 locations are those in which combustible dust is not normally present but might be due to abnormal or periodic operations. During those times, sufficient dust may be present in the air to produce explosive or ignitable mixtures. A Class II, Division 2 location is an area normally free of dust, but due to some incident, dust may be introduced. Mechanical breakdown of a valve or a break in a pipe are examples of conditions that would require an area to be classified as Division 2.

7) Answer C:
According to The NFPA Fire Protection Handbook, for combustion to occur, four components are necessary: Oxygen (oxidizing agent); Fuel (substrate); Heat (ignition); and a self-sustained chemical reaction (also referred to as the chain reaction). These components can be graphically described as the "fire tetrahedron". Each component of the tetrahedron must be in place for combustion to occur. Remove any one of the four components and combustion will not occur. If ignition has already occurred, the fire is extinguished when one of the components is removed from the reaction.

8) Answer D:
There are three types of heat detectors candidates should be familiar with for the examination. They are listed below with their general characteristics:
Fixed-Temperature Designed to alarm when the temperature of the operating element reaches a specified point. These units are susceptible to "thermal lag".
Rate Compensation Designed to alarm when the temperature of surrounding air reaches a predetermined level, regardless of rate of temperature rise. Element configuration compensates for thermal lag.
Rate-of-Rise Designed to alarm when the rate of temperature increase exceeds a predetermined value (usually 12 to 15°F per minute). An example of use would be on a petroleum-based hydraulic pump to prevent explosions.

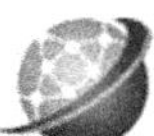

9) Answer B:

As described in Counter Terrorism for Emergency Responders, 2nd Edition, a chemical explosion, like fire, requires oxidizer, fuel, ignition, and chemical reaction but more importantly it requires confinement of the oxidizer and fuel. Without confinement, the materials will not explode; they will merely burn with great intensity.

10) Answer B:

According to the Root Cause Analysis Handbook, 2005 Edition, to gather data from people, the analyst must be a skilled interviewer. During the interview the interviewer must ask open ended questions that require the interviewee to respond with a long, descriptive answer

11) Answer A:

In the book *Root Cause Analysis Handbook, An Effective Guide to Incident Investigation* chain of custody procedures for photographs start with the photographer fully documenting the context, source, and relevant information related to the photograph.

12) Answer C:

Accident investigation has as its primary purpose the prevention of similar occurrences and the discovery of hazards. The intent is not to place blame or administer discipline, but rather to determine how responsibilities may be defined or clarified and to reduce error producing situations. Accident investigation should improve the safety of operations, if accident investigation is used for punitive measures, the tool has the reverse effect. Management system problems are unifying characteristics of root causes of incidents or accidents. Human errors and equipment malfunctions are the causal factors from which the root causes are derived.

13) Answer C:

In the book *Safety Culture and Effective Safety Management,* author Swartz explains that before collecting data and developing a system to collect and manipulate the data, it is essential to define how the data will be used.

14) Answer A:
You must always base your findings and recommendations on facts, which means that your first action should always be to survey the situation and collect the facts that may impact the situation.

15) Answer B:
The **Critical Incident Technique** (or **CIT**) is a set of procedures used for collecting first hand observations of human behavior that have critical significance and meet methodically defined criteria. A critical incident can be described as one that makes a significant contribution—either positively or negatively—to an activity or phenomenon and to understand the relationship between competencies and reasons for accidents. Critical incidents can be gathered in various ways, but typically respondents are asked to tell a story about an experience they have had.
Through the use of the critical incident technique one may collect specific and significant behavioral facts, providing a sound basis for making inferences as to requirements for measures of typical performance (criteria), measures of proficiency (standard samples), training, selection and classification, job design, operating procedures, equipment design, motivation and leadership (attitudes), and individual behavior.
Critical incidents can be gathered in various ways, but typically respondents are asked to tell a story about an experience they have had. CIT is a flexible method that usually relies on five major areas. The first is determining and reviewing the incident, then fact-finding, which involves collecting the details of the incident from the participants.
When all facts are collected, the next step is to identify the issues. Afterwards a decision can be made on how to resolve the issues based on various possible solutions. The final and most important aspect is the evaluation which will determine if the solution that was selected will solve the situation's root cause and will cause no further problems.

16) Answer B:
As described in *Root Cause Analysis Handbook, an Effective Guide to Incident Investigation. 2005* Edition, management system problems are unifying characteristics of root causes of incidents. Human errors and equipment malfunction; are example of causal factors driving the root causes.

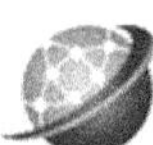

17) Answer A:

The publication *Process Safety Leading and Lagging Metrics,* published by the Center for Chemical Process Safety (2007) gives specifically related guidance on determining and applying leading and lagging indicators in the practice of safety. Three types of process safety performance metrics are described and the text on their selection and application is extensive. The metrics are lagging metrics, leading metrics, and near miss and other internal lagging metrics. The metrics pertain only to chemical process incidents and near misses, to the exclusion of types of incidents that are not process related. The leading process safety metrics given particular attention are: maintenance of mechanical integrity; action items follow-up; management of change; process safety training and competency (and training competency assessment). Companies should identify which of these components are most important for ensuring the safety of their facilities, and should select the most meaningful leading metrics from the examples [above], and where significant performance improvement potentially exists. Other leading metrics may be defined as well if applicable.

18) Answer D:

An incidence rate of injuries and illnesses may be computed from the following formula:

$$\text{Incident Rate} = \frac{\#\text{of Incidents} \times 200{,}000}{\text{Total hours worked}}$$

The 200,000 hours in the formula represents the equivalent of 100 employees working 40 hours per week, 50 weeks per year, and provides the standard base for the incidence rates. You can use the same formula to compute incidence rates for:

- Injury and illness cases with days away from work
- Injury and Illness cases with job transfer or restriction
- Injury and illness cases with days away from work, or job transfer or restriction, or both (DART)
- Other recordable injury and illness cases
- Injury-only cases
- Illness-only cases

"Hours worked" should not include any nonwork time, even though paid, such as vacation, sick leave, holidays, etc. If actual hours worked are not available for employees paid on commission, by salary, or by the mile, etc., hours worked may be estimated on the basis of scheduled hours or 8 hours per workday. Vehicle accidents are generally measured per million miles, whereas injury rates are figured per 200,000 work hours or 100 workers working one year.

$$\text{Fleet Incident Rate} = \frac{\#\text{of Incidents} \times 1{,}000{,}000}{\text{Miles Driven}}$$

$$\text{Fleet Incident Rate} = \frac{\#\text{of Incidents} \times 1{,}600{,}000}{\text{Kilometers Driven}}$$

19) Answer A:
5-Whys is a qualitative analytical technique to identify the root causes of an incident sequence by asking "why" at least 5 times. Once the causal factors (human errors, equipment malfunctions, etc.) are known, a 5-Whys analysis can be performed on each causal factor to determine "Why" the causal factor could exist.

20) Answer B:
The best place to interview a witness during an accident investigation is the accident site, if this is not possible you want a private location that will not intimidate, inhibit or distract the witness. Your office or a supervisor's office may be intimidating.

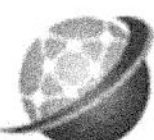

Domain 4 Quiz 2 Questions

1) A flood destroys a company's operations ability. After emergency management issues are addressed, the business implements several plans for recovery of critical files and information that had been stored offsite, establishes a temporary facility from which operations can be conducted, informs customers of circumstances and how customers will be served. These plans are examples of a comprehensive loss control activity called:
   A) Emergency Management/Emergency Response.
   B) Situational Awareness.
   C) Disaster Recovery/Business Continuity Planning.
   D) Business Impact Analysis.

2) Advanced emergency management planning is the best way to minimize potential loss from natural or technological disasters and accidents. The primary responsibilities of emergency planning must **exclude**:
   A) Establishing continuity of operations for the customers' sake.
   B) Providing for the safety of employees and public.
   C) Protecting property and environment.
   D) Establishing methods to restore operations to a new normal as soon as possible.

3) A number of different agencies might be responsible for controlling and cleaning up more complex hazardous materials incidents. Which is the **first** step in responding to chemical release when multi agencies are involved?
   A) Approve the Incident Action Plan.
   B) Establish the Incident Command System.
   C) Approve resource requests.
   D) Order demobilization.

4) The National Incident Management System (NIMS) is the responsibility of the:
   A) Department of State (DOS).
   B) Department of Health and Human Services (DHHS).
   C) Department of Defense (DOD).
   D) Department of Homeland Security(DHS).

5) Under ICS, the Command Staff positions include:
   A) Safety Officer, Public Information Officer, and Liaison Officer.
   B) Liaison Officer, Operations Section Chief, and Finance and Administration Section Chief.
   C) Public Information Officer, Chief Executive Officer, and Safety Officer.
   D) Logistics Section Chief, Safety Officer, and the Contracting Officer.

6) Which training level applies to employees who are only likely to witness or discover a hazardous substance release and who need to be trained to initiate an emergency response sequence by notifying the proper authorities of the release?
   A) Awareness Level.
   B) Operations Level.
   C) Hazardous Materials Technicians.
   D) Specialist employees.

7) The **primary** health exposure concern with removal of old paint is
   A) Asbestos.
   B) Cadmium.
   C) Lead.
   D) Mercury.

8) The general public resists change for all the following reasons **except**?
   A) Fear of the unknown.
   B) False confidence.
   C) Loss of face.
   D) Lack of purpose.

9) The **most** important spokesperson characteristics for effective risk communication to the public are:
   A) Expertise and authoritative presence.
   B) Appearance and empathy.
   C) Authoritative presence and credibility.
   D) Credibility and technical competency.

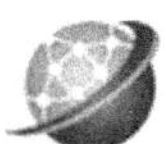

10) To effectively perform a job safety analysis, a safety manager should strive to:
   A) Identify every possible occurrence involved with the task.
   B) Empower the work team to compile the analysis and discuss it at the work location.
   C) Make certain it is signed by every team member.
   D) Use a consistent form and numbered work tasks for ease of use on every analysis.

11) The Incident Command System (ICS) recognizes that field response is where response personnel carry out tactical decisions and activities in direct response to an incident, under the command of:
   A) Federal Government.
   B) An appropriate authority.
   C) Local Government.
   D) Private Contractors.

12) The Management Oversight and Risk Tree (MORT) methodology generally focuses on which of the following concerns?
   A) Assumed risks, and Hazard Evaluation.
   B) Management Errors and Risk Evaluation.
   C) Decision analysis and Assumed risks.
   D) Oversights and omissions and Management system errors.

13) The primary reason safety professionals perform incident investigation is to determine causal conditions and identify preventative controls. The responsibility for implementing the corrective actions generally is the responsibility of the:
   A) Line Supervisor.
   B) Safety manager.
   C) Compliance officer.
   D) Site manager.

14) All of the following are valid reasons for accident (mishap) investigation **except**?
   A) Prevent reoccurrence of similar events.
   B) Establish casual factors.
   C) Provide vehicle for discipline.
   D) Provide data for trend analysis.

15) An structural mishap at one of the buildings at your plant has occurred and you have just been given responsibility for the investigation and for control of the accident scene. From most important to least important, which of the following best indicates the correct order of actions you should take?

A) 1,2,3,4	1.)	Arrive safely
B) 1,3,2,4	2.)	Care for the injured
C) 1,4,2,3	3.)	Size-up the situation
D) 1,2,4,3	4.)	Protect property

16) Employees experienced several slips and falls in a newly constructed area of a warehouse. This has been occurring for several weeks and the problem has finally been corrected by installing skid resistant material on the walkways. When should this problem have identified?

A) After the first incident.
B) By the company insurance "safety expert".
C) By maintenance personnel.
D) During review of the building design plans.

17) A company uses several temp agencies and contract workers. Data indicates an increase in incidents among this group of workers at facility. The **best** course of action is to:

A) Do a new more comprehensive contractor new hire orientation.
B) Implement and enforce a zero tolerance disciplinary policy.
C) Do nothing as these workers are not employees of the company.
D) Develop a contractor safety committee to discuss issues and solutions.

18) Which of the following is a tool commonly used in root cause analysis?

A) Fish bone.
B) Kaizen.
C) Job safety.
D) Soft tree.

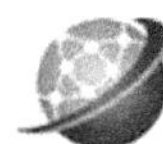

19) As part of a pre-incident investigation campaign, site observations indicate a decrease in PPE usage. Considering a PPE assessment has been conducted and required PPE is available, the **best** method to communicate the PPE requirements to workers is to:

A) Send an email to all the subcontractor company owners.
B) Conduct an all site meeting about PPE requirements.
C) Write the findings in the observation report.
D) Post the observation findings in the job trailer.

20) When conducting hazard analysis for newly purchased equipment, which resources should you acquire **first** to identify potential hazards associated with equipment?

A) A past history of law suits and insurance claims related to the equipment.
B) Benchmark data from companies who use the equipment.
C) Equipment manufacturers' product maintenance and operation manuals.
D) Regulatory agencies' reports of incidents involving the equipment.

Domain 4 Quiz 2 Answers

1) Answer C:

According to Risk Analysis and the Security Survey, 3rd Edition, business continuity planning is a key part of a loss control program. Such plans should include recovering corporate information, setting up operations, and financing temporary operations until a new facility can be commissioned. Depending upon the risk of a natural disaster, some companies purchase business interruption insurance to help finance operations.

2) Answer A:

According to the National Safety Council, advanced emergency management planning should include the following and they should be ranked as they are sequenced.

- Provide for the safety of employees and public
- Protect property and the environment
- Establish methods to restore operations to normal as soon as possible

When developing emergency management plans, sometimes the fundamental purpose is lost, which is to protect life, property and the environment. Though command and communication responsibilities are important and must be part of the planning process, fundamental strategies have to be developed to protect people, property and the environment and then tactics can be applied.
When developing a risk management plan, one must anticipate what will go wrong and make timely attempts to overcome identified loss scenarios. The risk management process consists of the following steps:

- Identify loss scenarios
- Develop alternatives to control them
- Implement best solution(s)
- Manage and control risk(s)

3) Answer B:

According the NFPA Hazardous Materials/WMD Response Handbook (2008), all of the answers are tasks for the Incident Commander. A vital step during pre-incident planning is to identify these agencies. The first thing to establish is the Incident Command System and designate who is in charge.

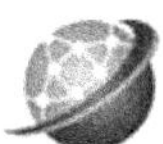

The National Incident Management System establishes the following functions as the Incident Commander(IC) primary responsibilities:

- Have clear authority and know agency policy.
- Ensure incident safety.
- Establish the incident command post (ICP).
- Set priorities, determine incident objectives and strategies.
- Establish incident command system (ICS).
- Approve incident response plan (IAP).
- Coordinate command and general staff activities.
- Approve resource requests and use of volunteers and auxiliary personnel.
- Order demobilization as needed.
- Ensure after action review.

4) Answer D:

The *National Incident Management System (NIMS)*, is the responsibility of the Department of Homeland Security (DHS). It provides a consistent template for managing incidents is a companion document to the National Response Framework and provides standard command and management structures that apply to response activities. This system provides a consistent, nationwide template to enable Federal, State, tribal, and local governments, the private sector, and Non-governmental Organizations (NGOs) to work together to prepare for, prevent, respond to, recover from, and mitigate the effects of incidents, regardless of cause, size, location, or complexity. This consistency provides the foundation for utilization of the NIMS for all incidents, ranging from daily occurrences to incidents requiring a coordinated Federal response.

5) Answer A:

ICS is organized into three components—Incident Command, Command Staff, and General Staff positions. Incident Command can be comprised either of a single Incident Commander or a Unified Command. An example ICS organizational chart is shown

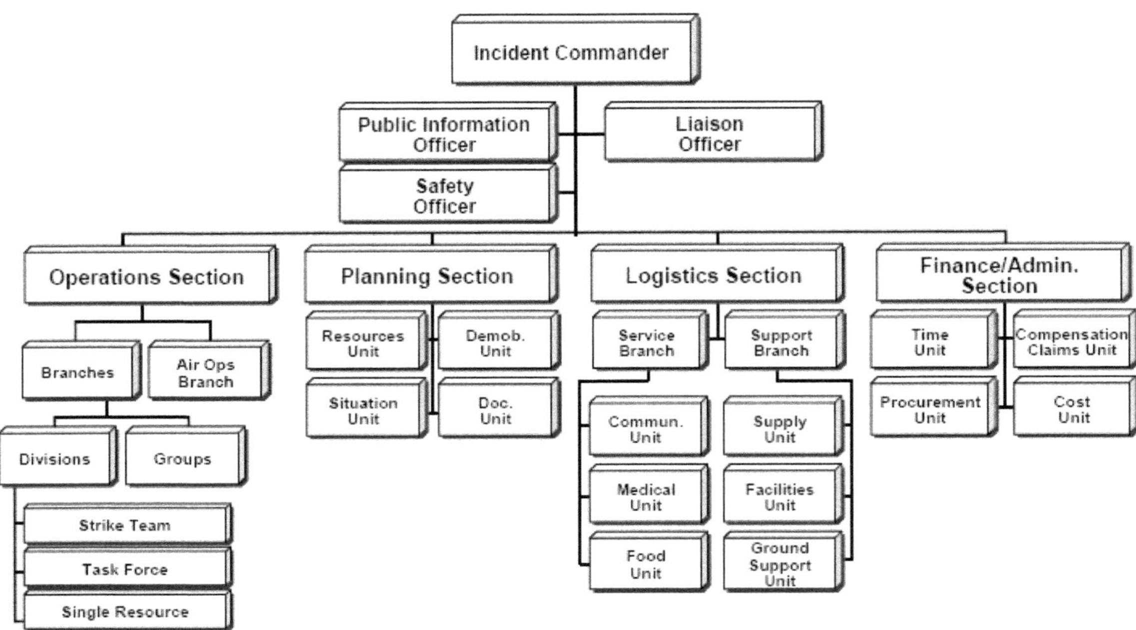

The Command Staff (CS) members perform incident-wide tasks and report directly to the IC. The three most common CS positions include:

- **Safety Officer** – responsible for the safe operations of all tasks performed on-site. The Safety Office has the essential authority to terminate any operations deemed to be unsafe, and even to override the authority of the IC to do so.
- **Public Information** Officer – the PIO is responsible for passing information regarding the incident to the public and to the media. Traditionally the PIO was responsible for press releases and public warning statements issued through the media. In recent years with the huge explosion of social media the PIO position has expanded greatly.
- **Liaison Officer** – this position is responsible for interacting and coordinating with other response entities not represented

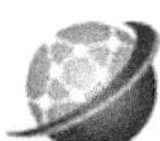

6) Answer A:

The OSHA 1910.120 HAZWOPER standard defines several levels of training for hazardous materials emergency responders. These include:

- **Awareness Level** - First responders at the awareness level are individuals who are likely to witness or discover a hazardous substance release and who have been trained to initiate an emergency response sequence by notifying the proper authorities of the release. They would take no further action beyond notifying the authorities of the release.
- **Operations Level** - First responders at the operations level are individuals who respond to releases or potential releases of hazardous substances as part of the initial response to the site for the purpose of protecting nearby persons, property, or the environment from the effects of the release. They are trained to respond in a defensive fashion without actually trying to stop the release. Their function is to contain the release from a safe distance, keep it from spreading, and prevent exposures.
- **Hazardous Materials Technician** - Hazardous materials technicians are individuals who respond to releases or potential releases for the purpose of stopping the release. They assume a more aggressive role than a first responder at the operations level in that they will approach the point of release in order to plug, patch or otherwise stop the release of a hazardous substance.
- **Hazardous Materials Specialist** - Hazardous materials specialists are individuals who respond with and provide support to hazardous materials technicians. Their duties parallel those of the hazardous materials technician, however, those duties require a more directed or specific knowledge of the various substances they may be called upon to contain. The hazardous materials specialist would also act as the site liaison with Federal, state, local and other government authorities in regards to site activities.
- **On-scene Incident Commander** - Incident commanders assume control of the incident scene beyond the first responder awareness level.
- **Skilled Support Personnel** - Personnel, not necessarily an employer's own employees, who are skilled in the operation of certain equipment, such as mechanized earth moving or digging equipment or crane and hoisting equipment, and who are needed temporarily to perform immediate emergency support work that cannot reasonably be performed in a timely fashion by an employer's own employees, and who will be or may be exposed to the hazards at an emergency response scene.
- **Specialist Employees** - Employees who, in the course of their regular job duties, work with and are trained in the hazards of specific hazardous substances, and who will be called upon to provide technical advice or assistance at a hazardous substance release incident to the individual in charge.

Each of these classes of employees must receive the appropriate level of training for the tasks they are to perform. The standard prescribes minimum duration of training and many organizations require longer training courses. Similar standards and guidance are provided from other sources, such as National Fire Protection Association (NFPA) 472.

7) Answer C:

Lead enters the body primarily through inhalation and ingestion and impacts the central nervous system. Workers can be exposed to lead in many ways:

- Lead itself is used on some electrical and elevator cables and on cast-iron soil pipe installation.
- Removing old lead paint and rust from bridges and other industrial structures.
- Renovating, remodeling, or repainting pre-1978 houses and buildings.
- Lead remediation.
- Lead solder is used in some industrial construction.
- Lead-containing mortar is used in some tanks.
- Pure lead and lead products, including lead panels (drywall/plywood), lead bricks, and lead shot, are used for shielding numerous military, industrial, research, and medical radiation sources.
- Stained-glass windows may contain lead.
- Lead use as a component in paint.

Employees may be exposed to lead by breathing in lead-containing dust and fumes at work, or from hobbies that involve lead. Lead passes through the lungs into the blood where it can harm many of the body's organ systems. While inorganic lead does not readily enter the body through the skin, it can enter the body through accidental ingestion (eating, drinking, and smoking) via contaminated hands, clothing, and surfaces. Workers may develop a variety of ailments, such as neurological effects, gastrointestinal effects, anemia, and kidney disease. A **medical surveillance** program includes biological monitoring for uptake of lead can involve blood lead levels (PhB) and blood zinc protoporphyrin (ZPP), which can show recent uptake. **Medical surveillance and monitoring verify exposure levels and the effectiveness of controls**. The hierarchy of controls describes the order that should be followed when choosing among exposure-control options for a hazardous substance. Generally, elimination or substitution is the preferred choice (most protective) at the top of the hierarchy, followed by engineering controls, administrative controls, work-practice controls, and, finally, personal protective equipment (PPE). Engineering controls include isolating the exposure source or using other **engineering methods, such as local exhaust ventilation, wet methods to minimize exposure to lead**. Administrative controls usually involve logistic or workforce actions such as limiting the amount of time a worker performs work involving potential exposure to lead. Good housekeeping practices to prevent surface contamination and hygiene facilities and practice to protect workers from ingesting and taking home lead are also necessary to prevent exposure to

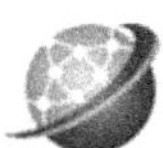

lead. When exposure to lead hazards cannot be engineered completely out of normal operations or maintenance work, and when safe work practices and other forms of administrative controls cannot provide sufficient additional protection, a supplementary method of control is the use of protective clothing or equipment. PPE may also be appropriate for controlling hazards while engineering and work practice controls are being installed. **PPE includes wearing the proper respiratory protection.** Employers are required to protect workers from inorganic lead exposure under OSHA lead standards covering general industry (1910.1025), shipyards (1915.1025), and construction (1926.62). The lead standards establish a permissible exposure limit (PEL) of 50 $\mu g/m^3$ of lead over an eight-hour time-weighted-average for all employees covered. The standards also set an action level of 30 $\mu g/m^3$, at which an employer must begin specific compliance activities.

8) Answer B:

A strategy to minimize resistance to change and drive ownership and involvement is to allow those affected by the change provide input during the change analysis. Some of the common reasons that people resist change are:

- fear of the unknown
- disrupted habits
- loss of confidence
- loss of control
- poor timing
- work overload
- loss of face
- lack of purpose

9) Answer A:

Spokespersons allow the public to put a face to the act of responding to, investigating, and resolving a crisis. How a spokesperson handles public and media inquiries, in addition to what he or she says, helps establish credibility for an organization. It also contributes to the public's transition from the crisis stage to resolution and recovery stages. An organization should carefully choose the personnel who will represent it.

The selection should be based on two factors:

- The individual's familiarity with the subject matter
- His or her ability to talk about it clearly and with confidence.

Risk communication (RC) is a complex, multidisciplinary, multidimensional, and evolving process of increasing importance in protecting the public's health. Public health officials use RC to give citizens necessary and appropriate information and to involve them in making decisions that affect them-such as where to build waste disposal facilities. The National Research Council (NRC) defines risk communication as "an interactive process of exchange of information and opinion among individuals, groups, and institutions." The definition includes "discussion about risk types and levels and about methods for managing risks." Specifically, this process is defined by levels of involvement in decisions, actions, or policies aimed at managing or controlling health or environmental risks. There are seven cardinal rules for the practice of risk communication, as first expressed by the U.S. Environmental Protection Agency:

- Accept and involve the public as a legitimate partner.
- Plan carefully and evaluate your efforts.
- Listen to the public's specific concerns.
- Be honest, frank, and open.
- Coordinate and collaborate with other credible sources.
- Meet the needs of the media.
- Speak clearly and with compassion

Factors Influencing Risk Perception

Risk perceptions more likely to be accepted	Risk perceptions less likely to be accepted
Voluntary	Imposed
Under an individual's control	Controlled by others
Have clear benefits	Have little or no benefit
Fairly distributed	Unfairly distributed
Natural	Manmade
Statistical	Catastrophic
Generated by a trusted source	Generated by an untrusted source
Familiar	Exotic
Affect adults	Affect children

Six principles of effective crisis and risk communication:

1. Be First: Crises are time-sensitive. Communicating information quickly is almost always important. For members of the public, the first source of information often becomes the preferred source.
2. Be Right: Accuracy establishes credibility. Information can include what is known, what is not known, and what is being done to fill in the gaps.
3. Be Credible: Honesty and truthfulness should not be compromised during crises.

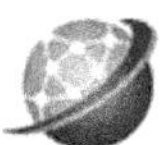

4. Express Empathy: Crises create harm, and the suffering should be acknowledged in words. Addressing what people are feeling, and the challenges they face, builds trust and rapport.
5. Promote Action: Giving people meaningful things to do calms anxiety, helps restore order, and promotes a restored sense of control.
6. Show Respect: Respectful communication is particularly important when people feel vulnerable. Respectful communication promotes cooperation and rapport.

According to FEMA, the person who delivers the messages plays a critical role in both risk and crisis communications. Communications experts have identified six traits of successful risk communicators:

- Communicator's speaking ability
- Reputation among audience members (trustworthiness and credibility)
- Subject matter knowledge
- Image of authority
- Obvious lack of vested interest
- Ability to connect, sympathize, or empathize with the audience

During a crisis or emergency, the messenger(s) puts a **human face on disaster response** and this person(s) is critical to **building confidence** in the public that people will be helped, and their community will recover. **Public Information Officers (PIOs)** regularly deliver information and messages to the media and the public. However, the **primary face of the disaster response should be an elected or appointed official** (i.e., mayor, governor, county administrator, city manager) or the director of the **emergency management agency** or both. These individuals bring a **measure of authority** to their role as messenger, and in the case of the emergency management director, someone who is in charge of response and recovery operations. The public wants to hear from an authority figure, and the media wants to know that the person they are talking to is **the one making the decisions.** Emergency management agencies should also **designate appropriate senior managers** who will be made available to both the traditional and new media to provide specific information on their activities and perspective. This is helpful in even the smallest disaster when persons with **expertise in specific facets** of the response can be very helpful in delivering disaster response information and messages. Any official who serves as a communicator during and after a crisis should **receive media training** before the crisis. Ultimately, communicators will seek to create **actual messages** that transmit certain knowledge, whether factual (awareness) or action-based (operational)

10) Answer B:

The majority of the benefits of a JSA come after its completion. However, benefits are also gained from developing the JSA. While conducting a JSA supervisors and workers learn about the job hazards. When employees are encouraged to participate in JSAs, their safety attitudes improve and their knowledge of safety increases. As a JSA is developed and refined, improved job procedures and safe working conditions are implemented more effectively (Hagan, 2015). The principle benefits of a Job Safety Analysis (JSA) are:

- Allowing the supervisor to perform training during safe, efficient operations
- Allowing the supervisor or other person developing the JSA to meet and work with employees
- Instruction of new employees on specific jobs
- Instruction of current employees on the specifics of jobs performed irregularly
- As an accident investigation tool should a mishap occur
- Studying jobs to determine if improvement is possible

When selecting jobs to analyze, one of the primary jobs to select would be the jobs with the highest accident rates. Job satisfaction surveys determine the employees' feelings about other departments, what parts of their jobs their feelings are focused on and areas of interpersonal difficulties.

11) Answer B:

ICS recognizes that field response is where response personnel, under the command of an appropriate authority, carry out tactical decisions and activities in direct response to an incident. For example, in a public established incident command center (ICC) in a disaster, the person in charge of the overall incident is the public incident manager. In a private company, the internal ICS a company incident commander would be in charge. ICS has fourteen management characteristics that make it useful when responding to a hazardous materials emergency (DHS, 2008):

Use of Common Terminology – Common terminology allows all responders unambiguous information flow. This common terminology applies to organizational functions of the ICS, resource descriptions (such a resource typing), and common names for incident facilities.

Modular Organization – The ICS structure is driven by the nature of the incident. While a full-blown ICS (involving perhaps thousands of responders at the largest scale) can be managed, the modular organization allows for

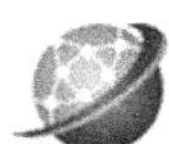

management of the smallest incident as well by staffing only those ICS elements necessary to accomplish the tasks at hand.

Management by Objectives – ICS identifies incident objectives through a planning process. All activities are performed in support of one or more of those objectives. Once all the incident objectives are accomplished the incident is over. Staffing of the incident is increased or decreased in response to the incident objectives. While not specified under ICS, it is always valuable to develop **SMART objectives—objectives that are Specific, Measurable, Achievable, Realistic, and Time-constrained**—as part of any incident action plan.

- **Incident Action Planning** – ICS calls for centralized incident action planning and only one action plan for the entire response. This ensures that all response activities are focused on the same objectives, improving the effectiveness and efficiency of the response.
- **Manageable Span of Control** – Every supervisor has a manageable number of direct reporting staff. ICS calls for a span of control of from 3 to 7 with 5 being optimum.
- **Predesignated Incident Facilities and Locations** – Incident facilities, such as the Command Post and the Staging Area, are defined. All responders know what takes place at each facility.
- **Comprehensive Resource Management** – One entity is responsible for tracking the status and location of all resources. This ensures that all resources are accounted for and put to the optimum use. No resource has the authority to free-lance or perform a mission they are not assigned.
- **Integrated Communications** – All methods of communication (radios, written reports, etc.) are coordinated to provide common situational awareness and interaction. A common communications plan and processes—including communications discipline—are integrated for the entire incident.
- **Establishment and Transfer of Command** – Every incident has a clearly identified commander appointed by the agency or entity with jurisdiction. If the Incident Commander changes this transfer of command is clear and transparent to everyone.
- **Chain of Command and Unity of Command** – The chain of command establishes the line of authority and decision making at an incident. Unity of command ensures that everyone present has one (and only one) supervisor. These principles eliminate multiple conflicting directives.

- **Unified Command** – In our federal system no one entity has all the authority necessary to bring an incident to a successful conclusion. Unified command allows those entities with some portion of the authority to pool their resources, if you will, and work together without losing any entity's authority, responsibility, or accountability. Typically, the Unified Command will consist of one representative from each level of government (federal, state, local, and responsible party, for instance) or geographic entity (adjacent counties impacted by the incident) to perform the duties of the Incident Commander, such as determining incident objectives and priorities.
- **Accountability** – Keeping track of all personnel and resources at an incident is critical to ensuring presence, health and safety, and responsibility.
- **Dispatch and Deployment** – Resources respond to the incident and are deployed only as directed by incident command. This reduces the occurrence of self-dispatch of resources and free-lancing at the incident scene.
- **Information and Intelligence Management** – ICS provides a mechanism for collecting, analyzing, and dissemination incident-related information and intelligence.

These fourteen elements make ICS flexible yet powerful tool for managing hazardous materials incidents.

12) Answer D:

The Management Oversight and Risk Tree (MORT) is a specific, detailed analytical method of evaluation of developing a safety program. It can also be used as an investigation tool to determine what is wrong with the accident prevention effort. MORT according to the developers Bill Johnson and Bob Nertney, focuses on three main concerns:

- Specific oversights and omissions
- Assumed risks
- Management system weaknesses

The system uses as a model an extensive MORT "tree". In practice the users of the system frequently use two sides of the tree:

Management Weaknesses (management factors)
Oversights and Omissions (specific control factors)

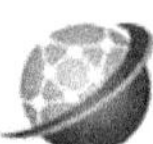

13) Answer A:
The cause factors discovered during incident investigations are normally corrected by the level of supervision that exercises control over the operation.

14) Answer C:
Incident investigation has as its primary purpose the prevention of similar occurrences and the discovery of hazards. The intent is not to place blame or administer discipline, but rather to determine how responsibilities may be defined or clarified and to reduce error producing situations. Incident investigation should improve the safety of operations, if accident investigation is used for punitive measures, the tool has the reverse effect.

15) Answer B:
In this case the initial actions, it would appear, have already been taken. Your remaining action would probably center on preventing a second accident and preserving evidence. However, in answer to the question, it is generally accepted within the health and safety community that the order of sequence for accident investigation should be:

1). Arrive safely: You cannot do anyone any good if you are involved in an accident yourself racing to the scene of a tragedy
2). Size up situation: The professional fire service uses the term "size-up" to indicate the time spent observing and analyzing the event. The same tactic should be used by investigators to determine what evidence must be protected, who is involved, who is on the scene, is the site now safe or is another mishap about to occur etc. Experience will allow you to accomplish this task very rapidly.
3). Care for the injured: If necessary the investigator should help injured and injured protect property. However, the investigators job is to gather facts not provide emergency service. Generally, this job is best left to others. It is fine to render aid if you are needed, but don't get in the way of the professionals. Protect Prevention of the second accident is an important property aspect of the accident investigators job. Because of their observation skills and training safety professionals can often spot unsafe conditions that others involved in the emergency will not see. You must above all else not allow an accident to escalate into a disaster.

16) Answer D:
Many accident producing situations can be discovered during the design review stages of construction thus reducing the time required to prevent mishaps.

17) Answer D:

The best course of action is to involve the contractor agencies and workers in a safety committee to determine the cause and solutions for the injuries. The need for employee participation is highlighted by several safety management systems, including ANSI Z10 (ANSI/ASSE 2012), OHSAS 18000, ISO 450001, and OSHA. Worker participation can take several forms:

- participating on joint labor-management committees and other advisory or specific-purpose committees
- conducting site inspections
- analyzing routine hazards in each step of a job or process, and preparing safe work practices or controls to eliminate or reduce exposure
- developing and revising the site safety and health rules
- training both current and newly hired employees
- providing programs and presentations at safety and health meetings
- conducting accident/incident investigations
- reporting hazards to upper management and/ or responsible parties
- fixing hazards within your control
- supporting your fellow workers by providing feedback on risks and assisting them in eliminating hazards
- participating in accident/incident investigations
- performing a pre-use or change analysis for new equipment or processes to identify hazards up front before use

ANSI Z10, Health and Safety Management Systems (2012) also specifically itemizes effective employee participation, including a role in activities such as incident investigations, procedure development, health- and safety-related audits, training development, job safety analysis, and all aspects of the planning process. In organizations where social responsibility is already a goal of the organization, the SH&E professional should already be able to identify several activities within the organization that address employee involvement. Areas where employee involvement is lacking or hampered can be more easily implemented by demonstrating that they add value to the organization's social responsibility goals. Examples of obstacles or barriers to employee involvement include: lack of response to employee input or suggestions, reprisals (supervisory and/or peer), or any other forms of discrimination (ANSI/ASSE 2012). Social responsibility is part of sustainability, involves employees in an organization, and gives them a voice on safety issues. Safety committee development is another way to demonstrate direct employee involvement in the safety program while also

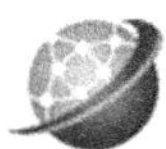

satisfying another component of good social responsibility. Safety committees are voluntary in many organizations but may be required by company policy or local regulations.

According to Petersen (2001), the least authentic is usually the traditional safety committee because typically only a few can serve on the committee. The safety committee structure can create a three-class workplace: management, involved employees, and noninvolved employees. This may create additional problems because the noninvolved employees must do the work while the involved sit in meetings. Although safety committees are traditional and they may be required by law in the future, they are perhaps the least effective route to employee involvement. Peterson advocates the use of improvement teams. Improvement teams are, in effect, ad hoc committees-people working together for a short period, solving a specific problem, and presenting their findings and solutions to management. Improvement teams can be ad hoc committees formed within a department because the boss has asked for help or task forces formed by upper management to solve a specific systemic problem. A team might consist of workers targeting areas like the following:

- ergonomic fixes
- identifying hazards
- identifying traps
- identifying systemic problems
- assessing culture

18) Answer A:

Root Cause Analysis (RCA) is a popular and often-used technique that helps people answer the question of why the problem occurred in the first place. It seeks to identify the origin of a problem using a specific set of steps, with associated tools, to find the primary cause of the problem, so that you can:

- Determine what happened.
- Determine why it happened.
- Figure out what to do to reduce the likelihood that it will happen again.

You'll usually find three basic types of causes:

1). **Physical causes** – Tangible, material items failed in some way (for example, a car's brakes stopped working).

2). **Human causes** – People did something wrong or did not do something that was needed. Human causes typically lead to physical causes (for example, no one filled the brake fluid, which led to the brakes failing).

3). **Organizational causes** – A system, process, or policy that people use to make decisions or do their work is faulty (for example, no one person was responsible for vehicle maintenance, and everyone assumed someone else had filled the brake fluid).

RCA assumes that systems and events are interrelated. An action in one area triggers an action in another, and another, and so on. By tracing back these actions, you can discover where the problem started and how it grew into the symptom you're now facing. RCA looks at all three types of causes. It involves investigating the patterns of negative effects, finding hidden flaws in the system, and discovering specific actions that contributed to the problem. This often means that RCA reveals more than one root cause.

Root cause analysis is a structured team process that assists in identifying underlying factors or causes of an adverse event or near-miss. Understanding the contributing factors or causes of a system failure can help develop actions that sustain the correction.

A cause and effect diagram, often called a "fishbone" diagram, can help in brainstorming to identify possible causes of a problem and in sorting ideas into useful categories. A fishbone diagram is a visual way to look at cause and effect. It is a more structured approach than some other tools available for brainstorming causes of a problem (e.g., the Five Whys tool). The problem or effect is displayed at the head or mouth of the fish. Possible contributing causes are listed on the smaller "bones" under various cause categories. A fishbone diagram can be helpful in identifying possible causes for a problem that might not otherwise be considered by directing the team to look at the categories and think of alternative causes. Include team members who have personal knowledge of the processes and systems involved in the problem or event to be investigated.

19) Answer B:

Safety meetings are a key part of a safety awareness program. Safety meetings are also one of the best methods to motivate workers and supervisors to improve safety performance. Safety meetings can be formal or informal and can cover a variety of topics. Formal meetings are planned and announced in advance to provide groups of employees with sit specific hazard information. Informal meetings, often referred to as "Tailgate" or "toolbox" meetings, can also be planned. These ad hoc meetings are often short covering a specific topic. These short safety meetings are very effective at relating safety to a specific job or work task.

Safety meetings are important to the success of your safety program because they impact all the following:

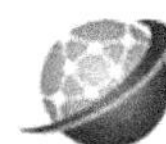

- Safety meetings encourage safety awareness. Other means of getting the safety message across are often too easily ignored. But, when a group of workers get together to discuss the hazards they have encountered and the steps they can take to eliminate them, it increases each worker's safety consciousness.
- Safety meetings get employees actively involved. In a sense, safety meetings put employees "spot on"; that is, they demand feedback. They get employees thinking about safety and encourage them to come up with ideas and suggestions for preventing accidents and minimizing the hazards with which they are most familiar.
- Safety meetings motivate employees to follow proper safety practices. Small group meetings are the best place to demonstrate the uses of protective equipment, proper lifting techniques and other safety procedures.
- Safety meetings can help to nip safety hazards in the bud. A safety meeting is the time to pinpoint minor hazards before they result in real problems. It also presents a good opportunity to discuss hazards that are inherent in the environment and that experienced employees are likely to take for granted.
- Safety meetings introduce workers to new safety rules, equipment and preventive practices. In addition to introducing new things, a safety meeting is a good time to reinforce the importance of long-standing safety procedures and to remind employees of the reasons behind them.
- Safety meetings provide vital information on accident causes and types. Regular meetings are the best way of keeping employees up-to-date on the hazards in their environment and what can be done about them. They also make it easier for the company to maintain accurate accident statistics, an important tool in tracing the progress of prevention efforts.

20) Answer C:

Product hazard information for equipment is usually available from the manufacturer. Manufacturer's recommendations for maintenance and operations are useful when evaluating tools and equipment for job hazard analysis, worker training, maintenance and inspection. Due to product liability claims, a manufacturer should keep product safety records as long as possible. Some states may have limits on time period, while other states do not and that is where lawsuits often originate. An example is the requirement of suppliers of services to attest that processes have been applied to identify and analyze hazards and to reduce risks deriving from those hazards to an acceptable level. There is precedent for having suppliers attest that risk analyses have been completed. Manufacturers of equipment to be used in the European Union are required by International Organization for Standardization (ISO) standards to certify that they have met applicable standards, including ISO 12100-1 and ISO 14121. In Process Safety Management, employers will need to review their maintenance programs and schedules to see if there are areas where "breakdown" maintenance is used rather than an on-going mechanical integrity program. Equipment used to process, store, or handle highly hazardous chemicals needs to be designed, constructed, installed and maintained to minimize the risk of releases of such chemicals. This requires that a mechanical integrity program be in place to assure the continued integrity of process equipment. Elements of a mechanical integrity program include the identification and categorization of equipment and instrumentation, inspections and tests, testing and inspection frequencies, development of maintenance procedures, training of maintenance personnel, the establishment of criteria for acceptable test results, documentation of test and inspection results, and documentation of manufacturer recommendations as to meantime to failure for equipment and instrumentation.

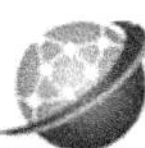

Domain 5: Business Case of Safety

Domain 5: Business Case of Safety 18.3%
Knowledge of: 1. Cost/benefit analysis principles and common techniques (e.g., return on investment [ROI], as low as reasonably practicable [ALARP], as low as reasonably achievable [ALARA]) 2. Direct and indirect costs in relation to safety 3. Experience modification rate (EMR), or premium rate, and how it is used 4. Principles of positive safety/organizational culture and common techniques for creating a positive safety culture (e.g., Hearts & Minds, behavioral safety management [BSM], behavior-based safety [BBS], stop work, open communication, culture or perception surveys) 5. Indicators of a positive safety/organizational culture (e.g., leading indicators, management system, management commitment) 6. Techniques and processes for communicating hazards and controls to stakeholders (e.g., management, workforce) 7. Presentation techniques or best practices for communicating technical and other safety information to stakeholders (e.g., management, workforce) 8. Conflict management techniques (e.g., situational leadership, good conflict versus bad conflict, diffusion techniques, relationship management) 9. Common leadership strategies or principles (e.g., setting good example, building trust) 10. BCSP Code of Ethics
Skill to: 1. Interpret cost/benefit analysis 2. Interpret leading and lagging indicators (e.g., training metrics, safety initiatives, incident and injury rates) 3. Develop a safety business case for additional budget, resources, other support, etc. (e.g., use financial tools to make a case for investing in safety program or initiative) 4. Communicate safety on multi-employer/contractor worksites 5. Facilitate or lead safety meetings (e.g., agenda, review safety plans, safety stand-down, shift handover) 6. Communicate (internal) safety activities and performance (e.g., reports, initiatives, lessons learned, requirements) to management and personnel 7. Communicate (external) safety risks and performance information (e.g., reports, presentations, risk/incident plans) to key stakeholders (e.g., public safety organizations, regulatory agencies, community) 8. Write communications that promote safety objectives and activities (e.g., safety proposal development, risk management plans, noncompliance response)

The Safety Professional

A ***safety professional*** is one who applies the expertise gained from a study of safety science, principles, and other subjects and from professional safety experience to create or develop procedures, processes, standards, specifications, and systems to achieve optimal control or reduction of the hazards and exposures that may harm people, property or the environment.

A certified safety professional is a safety professional who has met and continues to meet the criteria established by the Board of Certified Safety Professionals (BCSP) and is authorized by the BCSP to use the certified title and credential.

The primary focus for the safety profession is prevention of harm to people, property and the environment. They use appropriate methods and techniques of loss prevention and loss control. "Safety science" is a twenty-first century term for everything that goes into the prevention of accidents, illnesses, fires, explosions and other events which harm people, property and the environment. (ANSI/ASSE, 2007)

To perform their professional functions, individuals practicing in the safety profession generally have education, training and experience from a common body of knowledge. They need to have a fundamental knowledge of physics, chemistry, biology, physiology, statistics, mathematics, computer science, engineering mechanics, industrial processes, business, communication and psychology. Professional safety studies include industrial hygiene and toxicology, design of engineering hazard controls, fire protection, ergonomics, system and process safety, safety and health program management, accident investigation and analysis, product safety, construction safety, education and training methods, measurement of safety performance, human behavior, environmental safety and health, and safety, health and environmental laws, regulations and standards. Many have backgrounds or advanced study in other disciplines, such as management and business administration, engineering, education, physical and social sciences and other fields. Others have advanced study in safety, and this additional background extends their expertise beyond the basics of the safety profession.

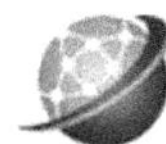

An American national standard sets forth common and reasonable parameters of the professional safety position in the ANSI/ASSE Z590.2-2003 *Criteria for Establishing the Scope and Functions of the Professional Safety Position* publication. Safety professionals must plan for and manage resources related to their functions. By acquiring the knowledge and skills of the profession, developing the mind set and wisdom to act responsibly in the occupational context, and keeping up with changes that affect the safety profession, the required safety professional functions can be performed with confidence, competence, credibility and respected authority. (ANSI/ASSE, 2017)

Safety professionals' precise roles and responsibilities depend on the companies or organizations for whom they work. Different industries have different hazards and require unique safety expertise. However, most safety professionals do several of the following:

- ***Hazard Recognition***: identifying conditions or actions that may cause injury, illness or property damage.
- ***Inspections/Audits***: assessing safety and health risks associated with equipment, materials, processes, facilities or abilities.
- ***Fire Protection***: reducing fire hazards by inspection, layout of facilities and processes, and design of fi re detection and suppression systems.
- ***Regulatory Compliance***: ensuring that mandatory safety and health standards are satisfied.
- ***Health Hazard Control***: controlling hazards such as noise, chemical exposures, radiation, or biological hazards that can create harm.
- ***Ergonomics***: improving the workplace based on an understanding of human physiological and psychological characteristics, abilities and limitations.
- ***Hazardous Materials Management***: ensuring that dangerous chemicals and other products are procured, stored, and disposed of in ways that prevent fires, exposure to or harm from these substances.
- ***Environmental Protection***: controlling hazards that can lead to undesirable releases of harmful materials into the air, water or soil.
- ***Training***: providing employees and managers with the knowledge and skills necessary to recognize hazards and perform their jobs safely and effectively.
- ***Accident and Incident Investigations***: determining the facts related to an accident or incident based on witness interviews, site inspections and collection of other evidence.

- ***Advising Management***: helping managers establish safety objectives, plan programs to achieve those objectives and integrate safety into the culture of an organization.
- ***Record Keeping***: maintaining safety and health information to meet government requirements, as well as to provide data for problem solving and decision-making.
- ***Evaluating***: judging the effectiveness of existing safety and health related programs and activities.
- ***Emergency Response***: organizing, training and coordinating skilled employees regarding auditory and visual communications pertaining to emergencies such as fires, accidents or other disasters.
- ***Managing Safety Programs***: planning, organizing, budgeting, and tracking completion and effectiveness of activities intended to achieve safety objectives in an organization or to implement administrative or technical controls that will eliminate or reduce hazards.
- ***Product Safety:*** assessing the probability that exposure to a product during any stage of its lifecycle will lead to an unacceptable impact on human health or the environment and determining the appropriate auditory and visual hazard warnings.
- ***Security***: identifying and implementing design features and procedures to protect facilities and businesses from threats that introduce hazards.

Safety professional's work virtually anywhere where people might be exposed to hazards and provide technical assistance in identifying, evaluating and controlling hazards globally. Because safety is an element in all human endeavors, the performance of these functions, in a variety of contexts in both public and private sectors, often employ specialized knowledge and skills. Typical settings are manufacturing, insurance, risk management, government, education, consulting, construction, healthcare, engineering and design, waste management, petroleum, facilities management, retail, transportation and utilities. Within these contexts, they must adapt their functions to fit the mission, operations and climate of their employer. Not only must individuals practicing in the safety profession acquire the knowledge and skills to perform these functions effectively in their employment context, through continuing education and training they stay current with new technologies, changes in laws and regulations, and changes in the workforce, workplace and world business, political and social climate.

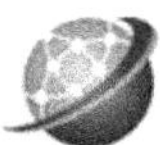

Professionalism, Ethics, and Codes of Conduct

Is it safe? How safe is safe enough? Who decides? Perhaps the most critical and frequently asked questions posed to OSH professionals. A primary role of the safety professional is to advise stakeholders and decision makers defining acceptable risk (INSHPO 2017, ASSE) and helping find tolerable solutions.

The art and science of occupational health and safety requires a dynamic mix of technical competencies and interpersonal skills. The philosophy of safety professional practice is hybrid of social and physical sciences. Together, "the art and science of safety" provide the professional competencies required to influence decisions impacting occupational health and safety. (Snyder, 2017)

Philosophy of Safety			
Philosophical Branch	Philosophical Focus	Speculative Question	Operative Question
Metaphysics	Study of Existence	What's is reality?	What is the perceived reality of the organizational safety and health culture?
Analytic	Study of History	Is there meaning in the historical process?	Will predictive analytics prevent future mishaps?
Epistemology	Study of Knowledge	How do I know?	How does communication training, education inform workers about workplace hazards and risk control measures?
Politics	Study of Force	What can I do?	How is decision making power influenced?
Logic	Study of Reason	How do I validate reasoning?	What evidence is needed to accept or reject hypotheses?
Ethics	Study of Action	What should I do?	Who is impacted by the outcome of this decision?

- Do we think differently when thinking scientifically than when thinking ethically?
- Can you find scientific answers to the questions "what is reasonable?", or "what is fair"?

A professional is defined as a member of a group of colleagues who have articulated a set of standards and values and can enforce them, at the very least, by exclusion from the group. Aim to show several different ways to think through a problem in professional ethics, rather than merely describe what professionals say are their problems (sociology of ethics). Professionalism can be defined as skill, competency in work. The ethical element is will the work be beneficial to others. Work itself doesn't have moral status, the execution of work has moral status. Professional ethics helps a professional decide when faced with a problem that raises a moral issue. The complexity can be many people, with many issues involved, the history of the issues and who decides, not just what is decided. (Strahlendorf, 2004)

Often use "ethics" and "morality" interchangeably but they are different.

- Morality – making choices with reasons
- Ethics – the study of HOW the choices are made, i.e. "ethics is the study of morality"

Ethics is a rational reflection upon good and evil (without weighing in on the question of heaven or hell, angels and demons). The word *ethics* refers to our identification of the "good" in any given situation as well as the rationale for the identification. Ethics engages each of us at the level of the thought, the reasoning process that goes into every decision we make, whether for our own happiness or that of another. Sound ethical judgment arises when proper habits of thought have given way to confidence in the right conduct and in doing it. As safety consultants (and mature adults), there is no flight from precisely this kind of deliberation. We should make choices that are responsible, defensible, and appropriate. Decide upon the highest good and order all the others, the lesser goods, in a hierarchy. This could be applied to a risk assessment or matrix. (Keys, Rodriquez, & Walaski, 2015)

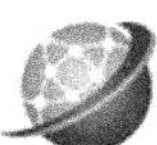

Reflecting on professional ethics and codes of conduct assist with choices about what one ought to do.

- Descriptive ethics – "What IS"
- Prescriptive ethics – "What OUGHT to be"

Codes of ethics require objectivity, which means that there are principles and values outside of the individual that the members of the community share and that individuals will be measured against.

There are rigorous professional guidelines and regulations regarding ethics for a safety professional. Below is a list of some of them:

- Board of Certified Safety Professionals Code of Ethics and Professional Conduct
- American Society of Safety Engineers' Code of Professional Conduct
- American Industrial Hygiene Association and American Conference of Governmental Industrial Hygienists Joint Ethical Principles
- American Board of Industrial Hygiene Code of Ethics
- International Code of Ethics for Occupational Health Professionals
- Federal Contractor Code of Business Ethics and Conduct (48 CFR 3.10)
- American Society of Civil Engineers Code of Ethics
- National Society of Professional Engineers Code of Ethics
- Institute of Hazardous Materials Management Code of Ethics

As a safety professional, you should be familiar with the codes of conduct pertinent to your work. However, in and of themselves, they are insufficient. You must also develop a robust code of personal ethics. The avoidance of wrong is not the same as doing right. As safety professionals, we must honor a high ethical standard, one that encompasses not just ourselves but our clients, colleagues, and community. You must not only behave ethically; you must strive to encourage ethical behavior in others.

BCSP Code of Ethics Standards:
HOLD paramount the safety and health of people, the protection of the environment and protection of property in the performance of professional duties and exercise their obligation to advise employers, clients, employees, the public, and appropriate authorities of danger and unacceptable risks to people, the environment, or property.
BE honest, fair, and impartial; act with responsibility and integrity. Adhere to high standards of ethical conduct with balanced care for the interests of the public, employers, clients, employees, colleagues and the profession. Avoid all conduct or practice that is likely to discredit the profession or deceive the public.
ISSUE public statements only in an objective and truthful manner and only when founded upon knowledge of the facts and competence in the subject matter.
UNDERTAKE assignments only when qualified by education or experience in the specific technical fields involved. Accept responsibility for their continued professional development by acquiring and maintaining competence through continuing education, experience, professional training and keeping current on relevant legal issues.
AVOID deceptive acts that falsify or misrepresent their academic or professional qualifications. Not misrepresent or exaggerate their degree of responsibility in or for the subject matter of prior assignments. Presentations incident to the solicitation of employment shall not misrepresent pertinent facts concerning employers, employees, associates, or past accomplishments with the intent and purpose of enhancing their qualifications and their work.
CONDUCT their professional relations by the highest standards of integrity and avoid compromise of their professional judgment by conflicts of interest. When becoming aware of professional misconduct by a BCSP certificant, take steps to bring that misconduct to the attention of the Board of Certified Safety Professionals.
ACT in a manner free of bias regarding religion, ethnicity, gender, age, national origin, sexual orientation, or disability.
SEEK opportunities to be of constructive service in civic affairs and work for the advancement of the safety, health and wellbeing of their community and their profession by sharing their knowledge and skills.

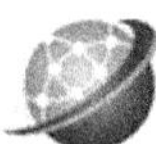

Program Evaluation and Continuous Improvement

According to ANSI Z10-2012, an Occupational Health and Safety Management System (OHSMS) is defined as a set of interrelated elements that establish and/or support occupational health and safety policy and objectives. The OHSMS should provide mechanisms to achieve those objectives to continually improve occupational health and safety. The illustration below depicts how the OHSMS requirements can enhance the approach to managing health and safety program activities. The circle in the middle of the diagram shows the OHSMS continuous improvement cycle based on the concept of "Plan-Do-Check-Act."

The management system approach is characterized by its emphasis on continual improvement and systematically eliminating the root causes of mishaps. The processes that drive the implementation of the organizational management system facilitates improved teamwork and operational performance. Establish performance objectives, especially for those issues with the greatest opportunity for safety improvement and risk reduction.
OHSMS objectives should meet "SMART" criteria:

- Specific—Clearly defined desired outcome
- Measurable—Concrete metric for success
- Actionable—Written as a concrete action plan
- Realistic—Practical in its scope
- Time-bounded—A specific timeframe is set

OHSMS evaluation and improvement involves continuous analysis of management leadership and employee involvement, hazard prevention and control, training and education. This may involve periodic review of program operations to evaluate success in meeting the goal and objectives. A comprehensive program audit is needed to evaluate the safety and health management means, methods, and processes, to ensure they are protecting against worksite hazards. The audit determines whether the policies and procedures are implemented as planned and whether they have met the objectives set for the program. This allows for the identification of opportunities for improvement and can inform the strategic planning process.

The success of an OHSMS requires a strategic map that describes major processes and milestones that need to be implemented and maintained to achieve a safe and healthful workplace. This strategy is intended focus on the process rather than on individual tasks. It is common for most sites to tend to focus on the accomplishment of tasks, i.e., to train everyone on a concern or topic or implement a new procedure for incident investigations.

Sites that maintain their focus on the larger process are far more successful. They can see the trending issues and thus can make system adjustments as needed. They never lose sight of their intended goals and tend not to get distracted or allow obstacles to interfere with their mission. The process itself will take care of the task implementation and ensure that the appropriate resources are provided, and priorities are set. An organization may use a qualitative or a quantitative evaluation system based on its size, operations, services, and culture.

An essential part of any safety and health system is the correction of hazards that occur despite the overall prevention and control program. For larger sites, documentation is important so that management and employees have a record of the correction.

Many companies use the form that documents the original discovery of a hazard to track its correction. Hazard correction information can be noted on an inspection report next to the hazard description. Employee reports of hazards and reports of accident investigation should provide space for notations about hazard correction.

Frequently, companies will computerize their hazard tracking system which can be as simple as adding a few items to an existing database, such as work order tracking.

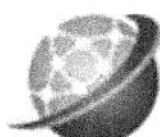

Objectives for measuring safety performance:

- Representative forms and procedures
- Information gathering
- Develop safe work practices
- Appropriate feedback based on data
- Documenting safety efforts
- Justify resources
- Stimulating prevention action
- Reinforcing performance improvement

Inputs to the Management review process may include:

- Progress in the reduction of risk;
- Effectiveness of processes to identify, assess, and prioritize risk and system deficiencies;
- Effectiveness in addressing root causes of risks and system deficiencies;
- Input from employees and employee representatives;
- Status of corrective and preventative actions;
- Follow-up actions from OHSMS audits and previous management reviews;
- The extent to which objectives have been met; and
- The performance of the OHSMS relative to expectations, taking into consideration changing circumstances, resource needs, alignment of the business plan and consistency with occupational health and safety policy.

Top management reviews are critical because they have the authority to make the necessary decisions about actions and resources, although it may also be appropriate to include other employee and management levels in the process. To be effective, the review process should ensure the necessary information is available for top management to evaluate the continuing suitability, adequacy, and effectiveness of the OHSMS. Reviews should present results to assist top management with prioritizing OHSMS elements. At the conclusion of the reviews, top management should make decisions, provide direction, and commit resources to implement the decisions.

100 Safety Performance Measures

1. Total workers' compensation costs	51. Vehicle safety audit
2. Average cost per claim	52. Fire protection audit
3. Cost per man-hour	53. Employee participation rates
4. OSHA 300 logs	54. Employee housekeeping
5. Industry ranking	55. Employee safety awareness
6. Behavior observation data	56. Employee at-risk behavior
7. Benchmarking other companies	57. Supervisor/manager participation
8. Employee perception surveys	58. Supervisor/manager communication
9. Frequency of all injuries/illnesses	59. Supervisor/manager enforcement
10. Severity of all injuries/illnesses	60. Supervisor/manager safety emphasis
11. Lost-time accidents	61. Supervisor/manager safety awareness
12. Investigations completed on time	62. Injury/illness cases reported on time
13. Investigation identifies causes	63. Statistical reports issued on time
14. Investigation identifies action plan	64. Ratio of safety & health staff to work force
15. Action plan implemented	65. Safety & health spending per employee
16. Safety meetings held as scheduled	66. Titles in safety & health library
17. Agenda promoted in advance	67. Technical assistance bulletins issued
18. Safety records updated and posted	68. Policies & procedures updated on time
19. Inspections conducted as scheduled	69. Wellness program participation rates
20. Inspection findings brought to closure	70. Security audits
21. Management safety communications	71. Emergency drills conducted as planned
22. Management safety participation	72. Percent employees trained in CPR/First Aid
23. Near miss/near hit reports	73. Absenteeism rates
24. Discipline/violations reports	74. Productivity per employee rates
25. Self-audits for regulatory compliance	75. Production error rates
26. Contractor recordable injuries/illnesses	76. Incidence of workplace violence
27. Total manufacturing process incidents	77. Incidence of accidental releases
28. Total transportation incidents	78. Employee exit interviews
29. Rate of employee suggestions/complaints	79. Employee focus groups
30. Resolution of suggestions/complaints	80. Community outreach initiatives
31. Vehicle accidents per mile driven	81. Off-the-job safety initiatives
32. Safety committee initiatives	82. Insurance/consultant reports
33. Management initiatives	83. Reports of peer support for safety
34. Respiratory protection audit	84. Certifications of safety & health personnel
35. Hearing conservation audit	85. Percent safety goals achieved
36. Spill control audit	86. Training conducted as scheduled
37. Emergency response drills	87. Safety training test scores
38. Toxic exposure monitoring audit	88. Statistical tracking for programs
39. Ventilation audit	89. Statistical process control
40. Lab safety audit	90. System safety analyses
41. Health/medical services audit	91. Contractor safety activities
42. Hazard communication audit	92. Positive reinforcement activities
43. Ergonomics audit	93. Compliance audit
44. Bloodborne pathogens audit	94. Conformance audit
45. Housekeeping audit	95. Willful violations
46. Job safety analyses	96. Serious or repeat violations
47. Lockout/tagout audit	97. Other-than-serious violations
48. Confined spaces audit	98. Total dollar amount of penalties
49. Machine guarding audit	99. Average time to abate reported hazard
50. Electrical safety audit	100. Average time to respond to complaint

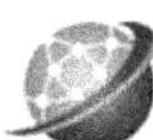

Performance Problem Characteristics

MOTIVATIONAL ISSUES	ENVIRONMENTAL BARRIERS	SKILL/KNOWLEDGE DEFICIENCY
• Individuals not in appropriate job for their training. • Individuals not getting clear/timely feedback on performance. • Punishment is a management technique. • Lack of clarity as to role in unit mission. • Good performance is punished. • Non-performance is rewarded. • Reward system is minimal or no reward for quality performance. • Tasks are distasteful.	• New equipment, system, or process present. • Required support equipment broken or missing from unit. • Work facilities inadequate. • Barriers to performance • Staffing shortages. • Work flow unclear. • Supply and demand difficulties. • Frequent supervisory changes. • High Turnover	• Individuals observed not performing a task correctly • Practice of tasks is non-routine or unrealistic. • Task requires the application of concepts, rules, and principles. • Task is new to job • A trend of inadequate training • Performance is complex and must be performed without using job aids. • Performance is guided, but the guides are poorly written. • Performance is poorly defined or described.

Below are some possible solutions to motivational and environmental problems, deficiencies in skills and knowledge, and flawed incentives and policies.

CAUSE	SOLUTIONS
Weak motivation	Information. Job aids. Coaching. Mentoring.
Faulty environment	Job redesign. New tools. Technology.
Absence of skill/knowledge	Training. Information. Job aid. Coaching. Mentoring.
Flawed incentives/policies	New policies. Management development. Supervisory training.

Ten OHSMS Strategies

1). Define safety responsibilities for all levels of the organization, e.g., safety is a line management function.

2). Develop upstream measures, e.g., number of reports of hazards/suggestions, number of committee projects/successes, etc.

3). Align management and supervisors by establishing a shared vision of safety and health goals and objectives vs. production.

4). Implement a process that holds managers and supervisors accountable for visibly being involved, setting the proper example, and leading a positive safety and health culture.

5). Evaluate effectiveness of recognition and disciplinary systems for safety and health.

6). Ensure the safety committee is functioning appropriately, e.g., membership, responsibilities/functions, authority, meeting management skills.

7). Provide multiple paths for employees to bring forward suggestions, concerns, or problems. One mechanism should use the chain of command and ensure no repercussions. Hold supervisors and middle managers accountable for being responsive.

8). Develop a system that tracks and ensures timeliness in hazard correction. Many sites have been successful in building this in with an already existing work order system.

9). Ensure reporting of injuries, first aid cases, and the near misses. Educate employees about the accident pyramid and importance of reporting minor incidents. Prepare management for an initial increase in incidents and a rise in rates. This will occur if underreporting exists in the organization. It will level off, then decline as the system changes take hold.

10). Evaluate and rebuild the incident investigation system as necessary to ensure that investigations are timely, complete, and effective. They should get to the root causes and avoid blaming workers.

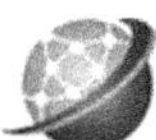

Domain 5 Quiz 1 Questions

1) A company representative visits a vendor to price some specific monitoring equipment. However, at the time of the visit, no purchase agreement is made. Later the vendor mails a proposed contract for the equipment and states that the offer is valid until July 1 and acceptance will be contingent upon a signed contract signed returned by U.S. mail. On June 15, a copy of the signed contract is faxed to the company. Is there a valid contract?
    A) No, an offer was not made and accepted.
    B) Yes, a fax can be used in lieu of the U.S. Postal Service.
    C) Yes, an offer was made and accepted before July 1.
    D) No, the acceptance was not as stated in the offer.

2) Define the term that indicates the product manufacturer is liable for injury due to a defect, without proof of negligence or even fault.
    A) Negligence.
    B) Strict liability.
    C) Privity.
    D) Res ipsa loquitur.

3) An employee was injured on the job and was sent to an occupational physician who ordered "no work for three daysthen return to work without restrictions." The employee's disability is called:
    A) Temporary Total Disability.
    B) Temporary Partial Disability.
    C) Permanent Partial Disability.
    D) Permanent Total Disability.

4) Employee unions can impact safety:
    A) Negatively when there is insistence for engineering control as a substitute for disciplinary action.
    B) Negatively when union leaders have a role in safety training.
    C) Positively when employees bargain for safety incentive programs based upon reducing accident rates.
    D) Positively when workers have more direct involvement in reducing workplace hazards.

5) Which is considered a direct cost when defining hidden costs of an accident?
   A) Time lost from work by injured.
   B) Time lost by fellow workers.
   C) Payment and benefits for lost time.
   D) Loss of production.

6) Catastrophe insurance is a low-probability, high-cost insurance against events that are generally excluded from standard hazard insurance. These policies for insurers are most closely related to:
   A) General liability.
   B) Business interruption.
   C) Reinsurance.
   D) Disaster liability.

7) The following are all criteria for evaluating cost-benefit analysis except
   A) The cost-benefit ratio.
   B) Gross benefits.
   C) Rate of return.
   D) Payback period.

8) A business has decided to implement a behavior-based safety program. What is the critical first step a safety professional needs to initiate in the process?
   A) Establish the data collection process.
   B) Develop the questions to be asked during the collection process.
   C) Decide how to codify the data once it is collected.
   D) Define the subsequent use of the data.

9) A company decides to reflect the worker's compensation losses against the profit function and to determine how many units must be sold to offset these costs. The profit margin of 2.5% on each unit sold and the worker's compensation for the last year were $90,000. What is the volume of sales needed to offset the worker's compensation losses?
   A) $ 600,000
   B) $ 3,000,000
   C) $ 3,600,000
   D) $30,000,000

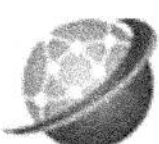

10) A steel manufacturing plant has a $1,400,000 payroll that suffers workers' compensation losses of $97,000. The experience modification factor for this plant is 1.6 and the annual premium is $88,000. What is the loss ratio for this manufacturing firm?
   A) 98%
   B) 38%
   C) 59%
   D) 69%

11) When a project has been proposed, it must first go through a preliminary analysis in order to determine whether or not it has a positive net present value using the MARR as the discount rate. The MARR is the target rate for evaluation of the project investment. What is the definition of MARR?
   A) Maximum Attractive Rate of Return.
   B) Minimum Attractive Rate of Return.
   C) Maximum Alternate Return Rate.
   D) Minimum Alternate Return Rate.

12) The **primary** benefit of an extranet is:
   A) Enhancing a company's intranet.
   B) Allowing information to be down loaded thru the internet.
   C) Providing accessibility to the internet by employees when offsite.
   D) Allowing secure admission into a section of business information or operations with suppliers, vendors, partners, customers or other businesses.

13) Padding the budget is considered a project budgeting method of:
   A) Marginalizing.
   B) Lowballing.
   C) Highballing.
   D) Estimating.

14) A systematic process for calculating and comparing benefits and costs of a project, decision or abatement actions is known as:
   A) Cost Analysis.
   B) Risk Management.
   C) Cost Benefit Analysis.
   D) Prime Cost Assessment.

15) In conducting a safety and health audit, an SMS asks for workers compensation cost data and finds the location's experience modification rate (EMR) to be 0.55. The rating for this location's safety and health performance based upon this value is:
   A) Good.
   B) Average.
   C) Cost neutral.
   D) Poor.

16) The Loss Ratio is defined as:
   A) $\text{Loss Ratio} = \dfrac{\text{Losses}}{(\text{Experience Modifier x 100})}$
   B) $\text{Loss Ratio} = \dfrac{\text{Losses}}{(\text{100,000 x Experience Modification})}$
   C) $\text{Loss Ratio} = \dfrac{\text{Losses}}{(\text{Manual Premium x Experience Modification})}$
   D) $\text{Loss Ratio} = \dfrac{\text{Losses}}{\text{Premium}}$

17) Accident costs and probability for the past year are reflected in the following table. What is the expected value of accident costs?
   A) $6,000
   B) $11,500
   C) $9,000
   D) $0

Accident Costs	Probability
0	0.1
$5,000	0.5
$10,000	0.3
$15,000	0.4

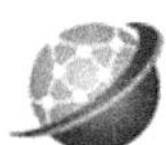

18) Two ways to modify insurance rates based on modifying the manual rate to reflect the insured's safety record are the prospective experience rating and the retrospective rating. Which of the following identifies the retrospective rating?
   A) Past experience.
   B) Experience during policy period.
   C) Projected losses.
   D) Manual premiums are not modified.

19) The management term "span of control" refers to:
   A) The breadth of a manager's expertise.
   B) The number of subordinates a manager can supervise.
   C) The number of projects a manager can supervise.
   D) The number of organizations a manager can supervise.

20) Which **best** describes the attributes of employee coaching?
   A) Achievement-orientated, reactive, fault-finding process.
   B) Achievement-orientated, proactive, fact-finding process.
   C) Achievement-orientated, reactive, fact-finding process.
   D) Achievement-orientated, proactive, fault-finding process.

Domain 5 Quiz 1 Answers

1) Answer D:
To be a valid contract, all requirements outlined in the offer must be completed.

2) Answer B:
Strict liability is the concept whereby the plaintiff need not show negligence or fault to prove liability. **Negligence** is the failure to exercise a reasonable amount of care or to carry out a legal duty so that injury or property damage occurs to another. An example would be you were a landlord and did not provide adequate security and the renter was robbed. In product safety work *Privity* is defined as "A direct relationship between the injured party and the party whose negligence caused an accident". A manufacturer or distributor would not have to label a large blade hunting knife because the product involves an **obvious peril**, sometimes called an obvious hazard that is well known to the public.
The term **res ipsa loquitur** (the thing speaks for itself) is involved in accidents where the damage producing agent was under the sole control of the defendant and the accident would not have happened if the defendant would have exercised proper control.
Foreseeability involves the liability for actions that a normal person would have known to exist and would have taken precautions to prevent.
Tort is a wrongful act or a failure to exercise due care that results in damage or injury in the broadest sense.

3) Answer A:
Most workers' compensation laws recognize four classes of disability: temporary total, permanent partial, permanent total, and death. Some states recognize an additional class: temporary partial. Definitions for and interpretations of each class vary by compensation law.
Temporary Total Disability Temporary total disability applies to a worker who is completely unable to work for a time because of a job-related injury. Eventually, the person recovers fully and returns to full job duties. No disability or reduction in work capacity remains after recovery. Most disability cases are temporary total cases.
Temporary Partial Disability This classification applies to injured workers who are unable to perform their regular job duties during the recovery period, but are able to work at a job requiring lesser capabilities. After recovery, the worker returns to work with full capability.
Permanent Partial Disability This classification refers to a worker who

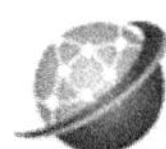

endures some permanent reduction in work capability but is still able to retain gainful employment. Examples of permanent partial disability include the *loss* of a body member, such as a hand, eye, or finger, or the *loss of use* of a body member, such as an eye, or permanent reduction in the movement or functionality of an elbow or other joint.

Permanent Total Disability This refers to a worker injured on the job and no longer able to work, even after medical and rehabilitative treatment. In many states, certain disabilities are classified as permanent total disability by definition. Defined impairments typically include loss of both eyes, loss of both legs, and loss of both an arm and a leg.

Workers' compensation laws provide payments for medical expenses, burial expenses, loss of wages, and impairments. Most provide payment for physical and vocational rehabilitation. Some provide for mental rehabilitation. Injured employees receive compensation for their loss of earnings, which can occur under all the types of disability. Most laws provide a percentage of the average weekly earnings of the injured employee. Payment schedules usually have upper and lower limits. Because disability income is not usually subject to income tax, a claimant receives only a portion of regular earnings. The percentage (commonly 662/3%) may vary by type of disability, number and ages of dependents, and other criteria. Some states limit loss-of-wage payments to a maximum length of time (usually for temporary total disability).

4) Answer D:

Unions are important participants in a safety culture. They want to eliminate injuries that harm their members. To do that, unions favor changes to the workplace that make it safer. Unions have challenged the reliance of some employers upon the discipline of individual workers for safety-related behaviors. Unions assert that the disciplining of individuals for errors is far less effective than a program of pre-incident planning, risk assessment, and engineering controls. A fail-safe device or design makes the errors less likely to cause injuries. The desirable investment in workplace design change that the union prefers would render the machine quieter, the floor safer, and the equipment guards impregnable to removal or evasion. This emphasis shifts the issues away from discipline of errant people to the needs for engineers to devise built-in constraints on peoples' capacity for accepting risk or making foolish judgments. In the event that work teams are used, the training of work teams for safety should include the support of union leadership such as the local president or shop steward for the safety program.

5) Answer C:

Incident costs include both those that are insured and those that are not insured. The insured include medical and compensation costs paid to the claimant by the insurance company. The noninsured include time lost by others who observed or rendered assistance at the time of the incident, time lost to investigate the incident, time required to train a replacement, cost for damaged materials, etc.

The term *incident* encompasses first-aid cases, recordable cases, restricted workday cases, lost-workday cases, permanent disability cases, near misses and property damage cases. Two basic cost categories are imperative:

a.) Direct incident costs represent actual cash outlays attributable to the incident; such outlays would not have been necessary had the incident not occurred.

Examples of ***Direct Costs*** include*:* Workers' Compensation; Medical-Related Treatment; Medical Treatment Supplies; Ambulance Service; Drug Testing; Job Accommodations and New Equipment.

b.) Indirect incident costs represent costs in terms of time and resources (other than cash) incurred as a result of the incident.

Examples of ***Indirect Costs*** include*:* Healthcare Professional; Injured Worker; Supervisor; Return to Work; Incident Review; Lost Production/Productivity; Human Resources; Cost to hire; Manager; Process Delays/Interruptions; Security; Training; and Legal.

Thus, total incident costs are the sum of these individual costs.

6) Answer C:

Insurance protects businesses and residences against natural disasters such as earthquakes, floods and hurricanes, and against man-made disasters such as terrorist attacks. These low-probability, high-cost events are generally excluded from standard hazard insurance policies, and so catastrophe insurance is required. **Catastrophe insurance** is different from other types of insurance in that it is difficult to estimate the total potential cost of an insured loss and a catastrophic event results in an extremely large number of claims being filed at the same time. This makes it difficult for catastrophe insurance issuers to effectively manage risk. Reinsurance and retrocession are used along with catastrophe insurance to manage catastrophe risk. **Reinsurance** (insurance for insurers) for catastrophic losses allows the

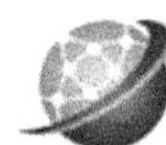

insurance industry the ability to absorb the multibillion dollar losses caused by natural and man-made disasters such as hurricanes, earthquakes and terrorist attacks because losses are spread among thousands of companies including catastrophe reinsurers who operate on a global basis. Insurers' ability and willingness to sell insurance fluctuates with the availability and cost of catastrophe reinsurance. **Retrocession** is the practice of one reinsurance company essentially insuring another reinsurance company by accepting business that the other company had agreed to underwrite. When one reinsurance company has other reinsurance companies partially underwrite some of its reinsurance risk, it essentially diversifies its risk portfolio and limits its potential losses as a result of a catastrophe.

7) Answer B:

The criteria for evaluating cost and benefits are:

- the cost-benefit ratio
- net benefits, benefits minus cost
- rate of return
- payback period

Not all costs and benefits can be converted to quantitative terms, some may only be expressed in qualitative terms. This can be the most difficult part of the formula. A major objective of applying cost-benefit analysis to safety is to provide a systemic analytical approach to dealing with complex issues of cost and benefit, assessing trade-offs in hazard control methods. Additionally, benefit-cost analysis is a tool to help management prioritize corrective actions. Though formal risk analysis identifies actions to reduce risk, a financial analysis is essential, so managers have the information to make judgments on how to spend money and expend efforts needed to reduce the identified risks by implementing corrective actions.

8) Answer D:

The first step you must always take when collecting date is to determine the use of the data and restrict it to only that use.

9) Answer C:

Since the profit is 2.5%, a volume of $3,600,000 is required to cover the workman's compensation losses.

$$90{,}000 \div .025 = 3{,}600{,}000$$

10) Answer D:

$$\text{Loss ratio} = \frac{\text{losses}}{\text{E- Mod} \times \text{Manual Premium}}$$

$$L_R = \frac{97{,}000}{1.6 \times 88{,}000}$$

$$L_R = 0.6889$$

11) Answer B:

This is accomplished by creating a cash flow diagram for the project and moving all the transactions on that diagram to the same point, using the MARR as the interest rate. If the resulting value at that point is zero or higher, then the project will move on to the next stage of analysis. Otherwise, it is discarded. The MARR generally increases with increased risk. The **net present worth (NPW)** is the difference between the present worth of all cash inflows and outflows of a project. Since all cash flows are discounted to the present the NPW method is also known as the **discounted cash flow technique**. This method not only allows the selection of a single project based on the NPW value but also a selection of the most economical project from a list of more than one alternative projects. To find the NPW of a project an interest rate is needed to discount future cash flows. The most appropriate value to use for this interest rate is the rate of return that one can obtain from investing the money. Alternatively, it can also be the rate charged if necessary to borrow the money. The selection of this rate is a policy decision. In engineering economy this interest rate is known as the **minimum attractive rate of return (MARR)**. In business and engineering, the, often abbreviated **MARR**, or **hurdle rate** is the minimum rate of return on a project a manager or company is willing to accept before starting a project, given its risk and opportunity cost of forgoing other projects. A synonym term seen in many contexts is **minimum acceptable rate of return**. For example, a manager may know that investing in a conservative project, such as a bond investment or another project with no risk, yields a known rate of return. When analyzing a new project, the manager may use the conservative project's rate of return as the MARR. The manager will only implement the new project if its anticipated return exceeds the MARR by at least the new project risk premium.

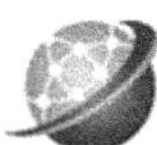

12) Answer D:

An **extranet** is a private network that uses internet protocols, network connectivity, and possibly the public telecommunication system to **securely share part of a business's information or operations with suppliers, vendors, partners, customers or other businesses**. An extranet can be viewed as part of a company's intranet that is extended to users outside the company (e.g. normally over the Internet).

It has also been described as a "state of mind" in which the Internet is perceived to do business with other companies as well as to sell products to customers. An extranet requires security and privacy. These can include firewalls, server management, the issuance and use of digital certificates or similar means of user authentication, encryption of messages, and the use of virtual private networks (VPNs) that tunnel through the public network.

The most common computer networks are peer-to-peer and client/server. Peer-to-peer networks are generally described as having three to five users (more than that can be confusing), they can share printers, scanners and fax machines and generally the workstations have the same capabilities.

Internets, intranets and extranets were created to permit communications among a variety of users and all systems are built using TCP/IP protocols, the domain name system and Internet Protocol addresses are the same on all systems and web browsers and e-mail can be used on these systems.

Local Area Networks (LANs) are a common means of making information available to multiple users. They consist of a network operating system that is specifically designed for transmitting data, communication links are both software and hardware designed to facilitate data transfer and Ethernet is a LAN technology.

13) Answer C:

According to The Safety Professionals Handbook (Haight, 2012), Once the decision has been made to pursue a project, the budgeting process should occur. A budget is a financial plan that establishes specific amounts of cash (and sometimes employee hours) that are expected to be spent on specific activities. Budgeting accomplishes many related purposes discussed very briefly below. Budgeting is a form of prioritization. By establishing a budget for a safety-related expenditure, one is securing management approval for this expenditure and is decreasing the chance that unexpected cash flow problems, or a manager's bad day, will prevent a planned safety expenditure from taking place.

Budgeting is an important part of cost control. Expenditures should be tracked and compared against expected expenditures for each point in time. Significant differences between actual and expected expenditures indicate either poor tracking (in that actual expenditures are not being assigned to the correct budget item), unexpected circumstances, or poor initial estimation and budgeting. This indicates that budgeting is part of the Plan-Do-Check-Act (PDCA) cycle of process improvement. Budgets are part of the short term operational plan. This plan is then executed as the do step. During operational execution, management should check by comparing actual expenditures to planned expenditures. If a significant difference exists between the two, managers act, resolving any unforeseen problems and, if necessary, adjusting future budgets to prevent future deviations from plans. Budgeting is an important part of decision making. A manager must estimate the costs to include in an economic analysis. This estimate usually forms the basis for one's budget. But decision making does not end once the budget is established. If actual expenditures significantly exceed planned expenditures at any time, it may be appropriate to reevaluate the entire project. How future cash flows almost always hold some degree of uncertainty means there is always a risk that the best estimates of future costs may be low. Most managers understandably want to reduce that risk by proposing a budget that includes a contingency amount; padding, but two problems arise when including such buffers in budgets. One problem is that allocating contingency resources to a budget prevents those resources from being used for other good projects. A second and even worse problem is that many managers will attempt to hide their over budgeting or “highballing” by inefficiently spending any remaining funds as the end of the fiscal year approaches. Decisions about budget allocation should be based on which projects will provide the greatest return on investment to the company. A process called zero-based budgeting has emerged to combat such budget inertia. Instead of each project or manager will receive approximately the budget they had previously, managers and projects are assumed to have no budget until they justify in detail why they should receive any funds at all.

14) Answer C:
Cost benefit analysis is a generic process of evaluating competing courses of action by examining the dollar costs of certain abatement actions versus the dollar value of benefits received.

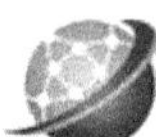

15) Answer A:

The experience modification is developed from the location's injury/illness frequency and severity rate and the industry rate and impacts workers compensation premiums. If the plant had the same experience as industry, the experience modification rate would be 1. Since this plant had an experience modification rate of 0.55, it would be considered very good.

16) Answer C:

$$\text{Loss Ratio} = \frac{\text{Losses}}{(\text{Manual Premium x Experience Modification})}$$

17) Answer B:

The expected value of accident costs is the sum of the costs times the probability of each occurrence.

Accident Cost		Probability		Expected Losses
0	x	0.1	=	$ 0
$5,000	x	0.5	=	$ 2,500
$10,000	x	0.3	=	$ 3,000
$15,000	x	0.4	=	$ 6,000
				$11,500

18) Answer B:

Because past experience modifies future rates, this plan is known as **prospective experience rating** to distinguish it from **retrospective experience rating**, which further modifies the manual rate to reflect experience during the policy period.

19) Answer B:

The well-known principle of "span of control" is defined as recognizing that a manager cannot effectively supervise more than a half dozen subordinate managers.

20) Answer B:

A behavior based approach treats safety as an achievement oriented process not outcome based. It also uses fact-finding versus fault-finding and is proactive not reactive.

Domain 5 Quiz 2 Questions

1) As a SMS, you are working as a consultant for a company and identify a condition that poses serious risk to the employees. You notify the client and he tells you that he does not have the money to fix the condition. The **most** ethical response to this situation is to:
   A) Report the situation to OSHA.
   B) Keep good documentation of this situation.
   C) Discuss the situation with the client to find a solution.
   D) You have informed the client and your responsibility has ended.

2) You are conducting a safety inspection of a manufacturing plant in the southwest and mentoring a graduate safety professional(GSP) intern. During the inspection an employee is observed, without eye protection, working at a bench installing parts. This is not a hazardous operation, but it is a posted "eye protection" area. Which of the following is the **best** course of action?
   A) Contact the supervisor and discuss the situation.
   B) Test the graduate safety professional skills to handle the situation.
   C) Confront the employee and determine "Why" eye protection is not being used.
   D) Send an email to notify the CEO and the supervisor.

3) The plaintiff's attorney contacts a SMS with specific subject matter expert witness for a highly publicized court case. The attorney offers to compensate the SMS with 5% of the settlement if the plaintiff's case is successful. The **most** ethical action is to:
   A) Accept the offer with an additional upfront retainer fee.
   B) Reject the offer and report the attorney to the BCSP.
   C) Counter the offer with an hourly fee schedule.
   D) Counter the offer requesting 10% of the settlement.

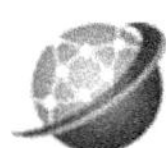

4) You are working for the general contractor and assisting sub-contractors with job safety analysis on a multiemployer jobsite. The Electricians identified a new Pipefitter task that would assists the Plumbers with installing water lines. The Pipefitters stated that the union agreement precluded them from assisting the Plumbers. What is the **best** course of action to resolve the issue of task responsibility?
   A) Assign the responsibility to all trades.
   B) Negotiate the tasks with the union representatives.
   C) Assign the task responsibility to only the Pipefitters.
   D) Notify the general site management staff to resolve the issue and communicate the policy to the appropriate parties.

5) A local safety conference planning committee has asked you speak about fall protection engineering on a construction safety expert panel. Your experience with fall protection is with maintenance employees in an aerial lift and cherry picker operators. You should:
   A) Attend the conference for professional development and decline to speak on the panel.
   B) Agree to speak on the panel only if the panel is not taking questions from the audience.
   C) Decline to speak on the panel and notify the BCSP.
   D) Do not attend the conference and avoid any conflict of interest.

6) Professional ethics refers to:
   A) A set of principles and standards that guide the actions of professionals that are often referenced in civil or criminal cases involving professional conduct.
   B) The laws that the professional must comply with or face possible civil and criminal charges.
   C) A set of bylaws established to assure the members of an organization must follow.
   D) Voluntary rules expected of members of professional associations.

7) Management has increased work hours and is pushing for more productivity. As a SMS, you are concerned about some of the safety risks associated with this production schedule. You should:
   A) Report concern to the US Department of Labor (DOL).
   B) Tell workers to launch a work slow down.
   C) Inform/communicate increased hazards due to increased. production and verify that risk is acceptable.
   D) Do not challenge the management; accept the production schedule.

8) As a salaried safety professional for a large company, you are obligated to be a faithful agent to your employer. You have recently purchased a substantial financial interest as a limited partner in a medium-sized safety consulting firm. Your employer recently acquired a new business that had hired your consulting firm to perform a safety compliance audit and you were assigned the task. After disclosing the conflict of interest to your boss, she permits you to perform the work. Is this an acceptable resolution?
   A) Yes, the conflict of interest has been addressed in accordance with your employer's code of ethics.
   B) No, because this situation does not avoid circumstance where compromise of conduct or conflict of interest may arise related to safety responsibilities.
   C) Yes, there is not a conflict of interest if the issue was fully disclosed to your employer.
   D) No, because the situation can cause you to be honest, fair, and impartial and act with responsibility and integrity.

9) You are part of an interview team to fill a new facility safety manager position. The candidate claims to be a CSP but is listed not on BCSP website as a credential holder, you should:
   A) Notify BCSP and give them all the pertinent information.
   B) Tell the person to stop using the CSP designation.
   C) Do nothing as the person if the person is qualified in other areas.
   D) Notify the corporate attorney to pursue legal action.

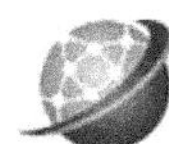

10) You are conducting an audit in a supervisor's area and he is a friend of yours. You identify significant hazards in his department, and supervisor tells you he will fix the hazards by end of day, which is best course of action?

A) Write it in the report and note the conversation with supervisor.
B) Write in report and noting the hazard was corrected.
C) Omit the hazard finding from the report since he said he would fix it by the end of the day.
D) Notify the supervisors boss of the hazard and ask her to verify the hazard has been abated.

11) Safety sampling is a management tool for making the workplace safer by studying how processes and people operate. These sampling statistics measure:

A) Accidental injury/illness performance.
B) Effectiveness of line manager's safety activities.
C) Risk potential for accidental injury/illness.
D) Job safety analysis.

12) In formulating realistic predictions of performance, safety professionals would apply

A) Trend analysis and past history.
B) Bench marking and trend analysis.
C) Past performance and diagnostics.
D) Bench marking and job safety analysis

13) The advantages of department level self-audits over corporate health and safety staff audits include:

A) Department auditors are more objective.
B) Department auditors are incentivized to reflect positively on their performance.
C) Department auditors can better assess problems they are most familiar with and develop feasible solutions
D) Corporate staff can differ to department self-audits and recuse themselves minimizing corporate bias.

14) The **best** illustration of a safety performance benchmark is:
    A) A thorough root cause analysis.
    B) Incident rate below the industrial average.
    C) Increased injury trends.
    D) Employee involvement.

15) In assessing a company's loss control performance, several key performance indicators (KPI) are collected and analyzed. One of these is "number of lost time cases experienced during the previous year." This dimension is an example of a(n):
    A) Leading indicator.
    B) Lagging indicator.
    C) Optional indicator.
    D) Occupational indicator.

16) How is a supervisor's safety performance activity measure best described?
    A) Reporting incidents to management.
    B) Classifying the financial impacts of losses associated with incidents.
    C) Initiating accident investigation on reported incidents.
    D) Performing safe work observations of employees and discussing observations with them.

17) A SMS must accept responsibility for their continued professional development by acquiring and maintaining competence through continuing education, experience, professional training, and:
    A) Monitoring safety websites.
    B) Maintaining a presence on social networks.
    C) Keeping current on relevant legal issues.
    D) Keeping a regular Internet blog.

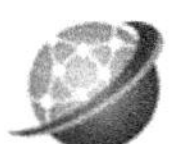

18) A SMS works with a large safety and occupational health staff. The SMS has been asked to perform hygiene sampling, even though the SMS has had no formal training or education on sampling. According to the BCSP Code of Ethics, what should the SMS do in this situation?
   A) The SMS does not have an ethics concern under BCSP professional conduct guidelines and should continue the sampling.
   B) The SMS may continue the sampling but should advise the BCSP that a possible ethics violation occurred.
   C) The SMS should perform the sampling but should contact BCSP after completion to verify if an ethics violation occurred.
   D) The SMS should not perform the sampling because doing so may violate the BCSP Code of Ethics.

19) The term *incident* encompasses first-aid cases, recordable cases, restricted workday cases, lost-workday cases, permanent disability cases, near misses and property damage cases. Which of the following represent an indirect cost?
   A) Incident review.
   B) Workers' compensation premiums.
   C) Ambulance service.
   D) Drug testing.

20) What is the **most** effective workplace communication method for critical or sensitive information?
   A) Mass email to the entire workforce.
   B) Place information in the company newsletter and send home with paychecks.
   C) Face-to-face individual two-way communication
   D) Post information on the employee information board.

Domain 5 Quiz 2 Answers

1) Answer C:
Your "first" responsibility is to try to get the client to fix the conditions. Hold paramount the safety and health of people, the protection of the environment and protection of property in the performance of professional duties and exercise your obligation to advise employers, clients, employees, the public, and appropriate authorities of danger and unacceptable risks to people, the environment, or property.

2) Answer A:
The first action is to protect the worker. Stopping the operation and discussing with the worker is most appropriate in imminent danger situations. In this case, you should be to contact the supervisor who has control of the workplace and discuss the hazards of the job and PPE requirements. Additionally, mentor demonstrated leadership by involving key shareholders and decision makers.

3) Answer C:
You must avoid the appearance of a "conflict of interest" to maintain your credibility. A flat fee schedule demonstrates that you have no stake in the case outcome. Conduct your professional relations by the highest standards of integrity and avoid compromise of their professional judgment by conflicts of interest.

4) Answer D:
It is important for a safety professional to realize when issues are beyond his/her control. For management/labor operational conflicts, it is best to direct the issue to management for resolution.

5) Answer A:
According to the BCSP Code of Ethics, certified professionals should undertake assignments only when qualified by education or experience in the specific technical fields involved. Accept responsibility for their continued professional development by acquiring and maintaining competence through continuing education, experience, professional training and keeping current on relevant legal issues. Issue public statements only in an objective and truthful manner and only when founded upon knowledge of the facts and competence in the subject matter. Not misrepresent or exaggerate their degree of responsibility in or for the subject matter of prior assignments.

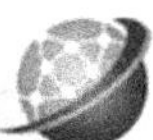

6) Answer A:

Ethics refers to a set of principles and standards that guide the actions of professionals that are often referenced in civil or criminal cases involving professional conduct. A basic definition of ethics is: moral principles or practice. Professional ethics require consideration of additional areas including, professional values, culture, acceptable standards of behavior and legality. Professionals will likely face ethical dilemmas during their career. Some day-to-day ethical dilemmas are simple to determine the correct course of action; others are not as clear.

7) Answer C:

Informing/communicating to upper management the increased hazards due to increased production and verifying that risk is acceptable is the best solution.

8) Answer B:

Most employer codes of ethics require you to disclose to your employer any conflicts of interest. Once you disclose the conflict of interest, your employer has the option to require you to resolve the conflict of interest by ending the relationship/situation that causes the conflict of interest or your employer can elect to allow the situation to continue. As per the BCSP and many other professional codes of conducts, certified professionals must avoid any perceptions of conflicts of interest even when their own company's codes of ethics are met.

9) Answer A:

If you have difficulties finding an individual or question an individual's certification status, please contact our office at bcsp@bcsp.org or at +1 317-593-4800. To report unauthorized use, use the BCSP complaint form. Individuals who have used BCSP credentials without authority are listed in the directory when you click the Unauthorized Use. The Unauthorized Use Directory is a listing of individuals who have claimed to hold CSP, ASP, GSP, SMS, OHST, CHST, STS, STSC, or CET credentials but do not. BCSP receives inquiries from a variety of sources including other credential holders, employers, and membership organizations. BCSP pursues all cases in which there is clear evidence of the unauthorized use and the individual has a clear responsibility, control, or knowledge of the use. Evidence may be a business card, resume, letter, web site, or other publication. BCSP may take a variety of actions because of verified and unauthorized use of BCSP credentials or marks. Such actions may include but are not limited to:

- Publish Name on BCSP Website: If it is determined that an individual uses a BCSP credential or mark without authorization, in most cases, a penalty will be imposed that includes publishing the individual's name in a directory on the BCSP Website and the period for which the penalty will be in place. If a person is found in violation of the Unauthorized Use Policy and a penalty is imposed, the individual will not be allowed to apply for, pursue, or regain the credential or mark for a period of five (5) years, or such other period as BCSP determines is appropriate.
- Cease and Desist Agreement: If a person uses a BCSP credential or mark without authorization, BCSP may consider an alternative resolution of allowing the individual to enter into a cease and desist agreement with BCSP. If BCSP determines that the said person fails to comply with the agreement the person will be subject to all penalties pursuant to the Unauthorized Use Policy and may also include civil penalties in the event BCSP is required to enforce the cease and desist agreement or take other action to protect its registered marks by filing a lawsuit against the person.

10) Answer A:

The best course of action is to note the hazard in the report along with the conversation with the supervisor with the planned corrective actions. The BCSP Code of Ethics states: BE honest, fair, and impartial; act with responsibility and integrity. Adhere to high standards of ethical conduct with balanced care for the interests of the public, employers, clients, employees, colleagues and the profession. Avoid all conduct or practice that is likely to discredit the profession or deceive the public. ISSUE public statements only in an objective and truthful manner and only when founded upon knowledge of the facts and competence in the subject matter. AVOID deceptive acts that falsify or misrepresent their academic or professional qualifications. Not misrepresent or exaggerate their degree of responsibility in or for the subject matter of prior assignments. Presentations incident to the solicitation of employment shall not misrepresent pertinent facts concerning employers, employees, associates, or past accomplishments with the intent and purpose of enhancing their qualifications and their work.

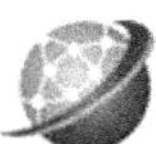

11) Answer B:

Safety sampling measures the effectiveness of the line manager's safety activities, but not in terms of accidents. It measures effectiveness by conducting periodic samplings of how safely the employees are working. Safety sampling is based on the quality control principle of random sampling inspection. The degree of accuracy is dictated by the number of samples taken.

12) Answer B:

A **bench mark** is defined as a standard or point of reference used for measuring or judging quality, value, efficiency, etc. Bench marking takes into consideration what is the standard for the industry and compares the status of your company in relation to reference point or data.

Trend analysis is the process of examining past performance for trends and then using these trends, or tendencies to make a prediction of what will take place under certain circumstances (e.g.; changes, modifications, presumed improvements).

13) Answer C:

The advantage of departmental auditing are involvement in the process and ownership of the solutions. Motivations for developing a management system audit program range from the desire to measure compliance with specific regulations, standards, or conformance with internal policies, to the goal of risk management. In practice auditing programs are designed to meet a broad range of objectives, depending on the needs of their various stakeholders. A Companies have established auditing programs to:

- determine and document compliance status
- improve overall safety, health, and environmental performance at operating facilities assist facility management
- increase the overall level of safety, health, and environmental awareness
- accelerate the overall development of S/H/E management control systems
- improve the safety, health, and environmental risk management system
- protect the company from potential liabilities
- develop a basis for optimizing safety, health, and environmental resources
- assess facility management's ability to achieve OHS goals

14) Answer B:
According to author Dan Peterson in *Safety by Objectives*, a safety performance benchmark is like a goal. A benchmark is based on research conducted on other similar organizations and applied to one's own organization.

15) Answer B:
Lagging indicators (such as historical statistics) provide data on how well the loss control system has performed and is useful for understanding how well a management system change affected loss control performance. However, lagging indicators are not as useful for predicting future loss control performance.

16) Answer D:
Author Dan Peterson explains that Activity measures are leading (proactive) measures a line supervisor should do as part of his or her normal responsibilities as being accountable for the safety of employees. *Techniques of Safety Management: A Systems Approach.* 4th Edition.

17) Answer C:
According to the BCSP Code of Ethics, a SMS should accept responsibility for their continued professional development by acquiring and maintaining competence through continuing education, experience, professional training and keeping current on relevant legal issues.

18) Answer D:
According to the BCSP Code of Ethics, a SMS should undertake assignments only when qualified by education or experience in the specific technical fields involved. UNDERTAKE assignments only when qualified by education or experience in the specific technical fields involved. Accept responsibility for their continued professional development by acquiring and maintaining competence through continuing education, experience, professional training and keeping current on relevant legal issues.

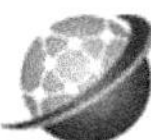

19) Answer A:

Direct Cost Category	Example
Workers' Compensation	WC premiums
Medical Bills	Treatment by physician, nurse, hospital costs
Medical Treatment Supplies	Bandages, splints, antiseptic
Ambulance Service	Established fees
Drug Testing	Fees for off-site testing
Job Accommodations	Equipment or tool redesign or replacement; ergonomically designed chairs, keyboards
New Equipment	Costs of new equipment/parts purchased as a result of an incident
Indirect Cost Category:	**Examples**
Healthcare Professional	Consultation with the victim; treatment time; recordkeeping and filing; follow-up consultation(s).
Injured Worker	All time spent away from the job attributable to the incident. One way to determine this is to ask the nurse or supervisor. Be sure to include travel time to/from the nurse's office, waiting time, treatment and follow-up, and time spent visiting the offsite doctor's office. An important, yet often overlooked contribution to indirect cost estimates is the percent reduction in efficiency due to restricted work. Often, an injured worker can return to the job at 100 percent; occasionally, however, the worker is only able to work at 90 percent until fully recovered. Once the percentage of restricted work has been determined, it can be incorporated into the indirect cost summary. Example: Hourly rate = $10; cumulative time lost due to incident = 2 hours. This yields an initial $20 indirect cost. Restricted work efficiency level = 90 percent for 8 hours. Since $10 x 0.9 yields work at a level of only $9/hour, there is a $1/hour indirect loss for each hour worked at the restricted level. Therefore, that $1/hour x 8 hours yields an additional $8 loss, which should be added to the original $20 calculation; thus, the ultimate indirect cost is $28.

Indirect Cost Category:	Examples
Supervisor	Consultation with the victim; recordkeeping and filing; follow-up consultation; disciplinary action.
Return to Work	Consultation, work process modifications.
Lost Production/Productivity	Lost production represents the expected income that would have been received from maintaining production/service that was lost and is attributable to the incident. Often, this cost amounts to the highest of all indirect costs. Also consider the lost productivity of witnesses and colleagues in discussing and investigating the incident.
Incident Review	Sum hourly rates of the incident investigation team, multiply by the average time needed to complete a thorough investigation for each cost category.
Human Resources	Managing the case back to 100-percent duty, consultation, recordkeeping and filing.
Cost to Hire	The cost in terms of all necessary activities to bring in a replacement employee to work while the injured employee recovers.
Manager	Consultation with the victim; recordkeeping and filing; follow-up consultation; disciplinary action.
Process Delays/Interruptions	Represents lost income expected or lost personnel productivity when a process is delayed or interrupted as the result of an incident.
Security	Since security is not involved in all cases, one must first determine the percentage of involvement. Example: Assume 900 cases occur and security is involved in 10 percent (or 90) of them. 90 cases x 1 hour of time devoted x $10/hour = $900 for all cases worked on. If security contributes $900 to the total, the cost for 900 cases = $900/900 = $1 contribution per case.
Training	Include new or retraining efforts, instructor costs, paperwork, recordkeeping and tracking. For new/retrained employees on a new job, one can also perform an efficiency analysis similar to that of an injured worker (see above).
Legal	Calculate same as security costs.

Labelle, J. E. (2000) *What do Accidents Truly Cost?* Professional Safety, ASSE April 2000

20) Answer C:

Face-to-face meetings with employees are one of the best ways to relay sensitive information. During layoffs or restructuring or when handling employee performance issues, face-to-face communication is generally preferred.

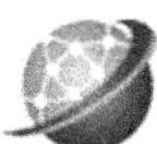

Domain 5 Quiz 3 Questions

1) Leadership styles can be dependent on the situation or team being led. In a situation where the leader is highly accountable for a task but has a distant relationship with the team performing the task, the **best** situational leadership style is:
   A) Selling.
   B) Participating.
   C) Telling.
   D) Delegating.

2) A safety culture is:
   A) The common and generally accepted way people behave in the workplace as it relates to safe practices.
   B) Defined by printed safety rules and posted signs.
   C) Described in negotiated agreements between unionized workers and management.
   D) Determined by the attitude that workers display each day.

3) A staff safety specialist is given authority by the General Manager to stop operations on a construction site whenever an imminent danger situation becomes evident. Which of the following correctly identifies the authority granted by the General Manager?
   A) Staff authority.
   B) Staff to line authority.
   C) Authority of delegation.
   D) Functional authority.

4) In the basic study of behavioral science, the theory of human needs by Abraham Maslow is often cited. In Maslow's theory a need is a deficiency a person feels the compulsion to satisfy. Central to this theory is the progressive principle, that is, the needs are arranged in a hierarchy whereby only after a lower level need is satisfied can the next highest level become active. Which of the following needs are at the **lowest** level in Maslow's hierarchy?
   A) Esteem.
   B) Social.
   C) Physiological.
   D) Safety.

5) Which of the following is the correct interpretation of this Pareto diagram?

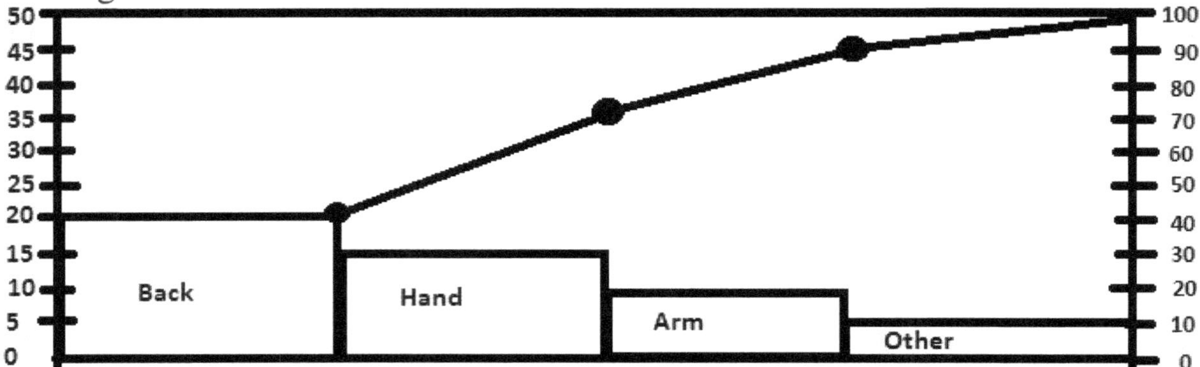

A) Backs represent 20 per cent of injuries.
B) The combined number of hand and arm injuries equals 30.
C) Knee injuries account for 10 per cent of injuries.
D) Back and hand account for 70% of all injuries.

6) Which of the following techniques is true concerning the *"Pre and Post testing"* method?

A) Pre and Post tests should be identical.
B) Pre and Post tests should not be used.
C) Pre and Post tests should cover the same objectives.
D) Pre and Post tests should cover different objectives.

7) A recent perception survey shows a significant difference in scores from labor and management on the topic of discipline. All other survey responses indicated perception alignment between management and labor. What actions should be taken based on this data?

A) Change the company disciplinary policy to be fair and impartial.
B) Conduct training on the companies discipline policy.
C) Management should further investigate the cause of the discrepancy in the data.
D) No action is required, labor receives the discipline and perceives it differently than managers

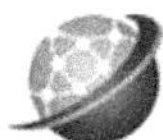

8) Which of the following is **not** integral to the development an effective safety culture?
   A) Safety managers must directly control worker behavior.
   B) Front-line supervisors initiate corrective measures for unsafe behaviors.
   C) Employees desire to be safe and work as a team.
   D) Unions take responsibility for ensuring safety as part of their role in protecting members.

9) The behavioral management safety concept is often criticized as dealing exclusively with behavioral modification. The major flaw in this view of behavioral based safety management is that it overlooks the fact that behavioral safety also plays a key role in:
   A) Securing management involvement.
   B) Establishing employee participation in the planning process.
   C) Identifying behavioral aspects of design and engineering for facilities, tools and equipment.
   D) Establishing a response loop for observers to report the status of safe and unsafe actions.

10) According to current safety philosophy, which would have the most impact on modifying safety performance?
   A) A sign stating "Wear Your Eye Protection".
   B) Turning off all machines when finished.
   C) Complementing an employee for wearing eye protection.
   D) A free meal for a safe month on the plant floor.

11) Which of the following factors is a hygiene factor as opposed to a motivation factor, according to the work of Frederick Herzberg?
   A) Money.
   B) Recognition.
   C) Responsibility.
   D) Achievement.

12) Which of the following would be most unsuitable for a supervisor when evaluating a subordinate during an annual employee performance report cycle?
   A) Offering advice about safety performance.
   B) Counseling about personal hygiene habits that affect job performance.
   C) Rating performance based on measurable objective criteria.
   D) Providing definitive comments about the worker's potential to fail in industry or business.

13) The definition of benchmarking is stated as:
   A) Developing predictions based on past performance.
   B) A process of comparing business processes and performance metrics to industry best practices.
   C) Setting standards in order to predict profits.
   D) Setting standards for rest of industry, so that operation can be considered superior.

14) A determination of the extent to which program operations have contributed to achieving an objective related to accident or injury reduction is called a(n)
   A) Effectiveness evaluation.
   B) General evaluation.
   C) Procedural evaluation.
   D) Administrative evaluation.

15) Organizations with effective safety management systems firmly assign accountability for safety to:
   A) Hourly workers level.
   B) Line managers at every level.
   C) The senior executive level.
   D) The company owner level.

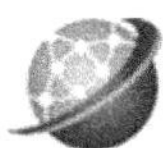

16) The Management Grid® by Robert Blake and Jane Mouton, illustrates management styles by drawing a grid which has on the "Y" axis Concern for People and the "X" axis concern for production. Thus a 9,1 supervisor could be called a
   A) Country club manager.
   B) Dictator.
   C) Workaholic.
   D) Company man.

17) When applying TQM techniques, the concept of empowering the worker frequently surfaces as a foundational issue. Which of the following is **not** considered to be a strategy of empowerment?
   A) Allow employees ownership of a tasking.
   B) Demand teams own the problem.
   C) Delegate authority to the lowest possible level.
   D) Develop rigorous procedure for multi-level review of team recommendations.

18) A company has adopted OHSAS 18001 to maintain continuous improvement in their safety and health management system. Based on the OHSAS 18001 guidelines that the management system should be suitable, adequate and effective, which of the following should indicate that a management appraisal should be performed?
   A) Earnings are down from the preceding year.
   B) SH&S Director position has been held by three different individuals during the past 18 months.
   C) A company's environmental performance has been questioned by the local "green" group.
   D) The safety performance of a company is 43% lower than the previous year.

19) Safety, Environmental and Health performance is best presented to upper management in terms of:
   A) Lost Workday Incident Rate.
   B) Total fatalities.
   C) Total lost time.
   D) Cost relationships.

20) Which of the following are used to adjust Worker's Compensation Insurance Rates?
   A) Experience Modification Rate.
   B) Incident Rate.
   C) Worker's Compensation Mod Rate.
   D) Accident Rate.

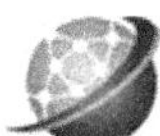

Domain 5 Quiz 3 Answers

1) Answer C:

The concept of situational leadership is leaders changing and adjusting their style to fit the situation and the people involved. Situational leadership is a well-established model built around the concept that each situation requires the application of a combination of two possible behavior dimensions-task or directive behavior and relationship or supportive behavior. In each case, a leader has to determine which combination is required by the situation and then correctly apply the appropriate behavior to properly manage the situation. They use four situations to describe the fundamentals of their model:

- Situation 1 (S1): High task, low relationship leader assumes telling role
- Situation 2 (S2): High task, high relationship leader assumes selling role
- Situation 3 (S3): High relationship, low task leader assumes participating role
- Situation 4 (S4): Low relationship, low task leader assumes delegating role

In an S1 situation, subordinates are usually new to a task and do not know how to do it. At this stage they don't know what they don't know. They need to be told what the task is and how to do it. They don't necessarily need a close relationship with the leader. In an S2 situation, workers are thought to be developing some competence, and now at least they know what they don't know. Because of this, they begin to develop more of an interest but still have to rely on the leader for guidance, so the need for a closer relationship is there. Developing workers want to know what the leader knows. In an S3 situation, workers have developed confidence and competence. They can handle the situation or task without input (task direction is not necessary); however, it is, figuratively speaking, the first time on their own, so they would like input and feedback about their performance and need a close (or high) relationship with the leader. In S4 situations, workers are fully developed and know how to handle the situation or perform the task without input and do not need feedback. Task-direction need and relationship with the leader are both low. A leader must be able to constantly assess this very dynamic process and correctly determine in which of these four categories workers or situations are. (Haight. 2012).

2) Answer A:
Making a safety culture successful is a real challenge for which the safety professional will need to invest time and energy. A culture is the way a group of people ordinarily behave, a common practice, like a culture of wearing casual clothes or dresses and suits. A safety culture means, in simplest terms, the common and generally accepted way people behave in the workplace, as it relates to safe behavior. The culture is a group's feeling that everyone has to cooperate for safety, and that everyone in the group will try to behave in a way that protects the safety of each other. If the workers believe in safety for themselves and others and then they act like safety matters in their everyday work, that is a workplace that has an active "safety culture." (Hagan, Montgomery, O'Reilly 2009)

3) Answer D:
The operational control delegated the safety engineer to shut down dangerous jobs by the General Manager is functional or line authority. This authority, or lack of it, is hotly debated by safety and health professionals. One position calls the delegation of such power unnecessary.
This opinion states that even the threat of a shutdown is most certainly going to be a confrontational issue. This is an issue that will eventually have to be resolved by higher authority and that often leads to long lasting negative relations between staff and operations. The other side of this debate believes they need the reserve strength over line managers because of the conflict between organizational demands and safety concerns. They further advance the argument by noting that the act of delegation of authority is a strong commitment by senior management to the safety process.
In many studies the authority of the safety professional has been linked to accident experience. Since the job is usually of a staff nature, the authority is often subtle. It is most effectively derived if the safety professional enjoys the confidence of a major executive. Another term that is used is "extensio", which is Latin for the state of being extended or the General Manager's authority has been extended to the Safety Professional.

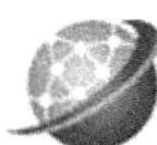

4) Answer C:

At the bottom of Maslow's "Hierarchy of Human Needs" are the physiological or survival needs of food, water and physical well-being. According to the *progression principle,* as soon as these survival needs are met, one attempts to satisfy the next level of needs; those of, security, protection and stability in day-to-day life activities. If these are met, one moves on to social needs. The first three needs in the model are called lower order needs and are concerns for a person's desire for social and physical well-being. The top two needs in the pyramid are the high order needs that satisfy psychological development and growth. Maslow's needs are often used as the most elementary model in the complex study of man's needs and desires. The chart below shows how needs are satisfied in life and in business.

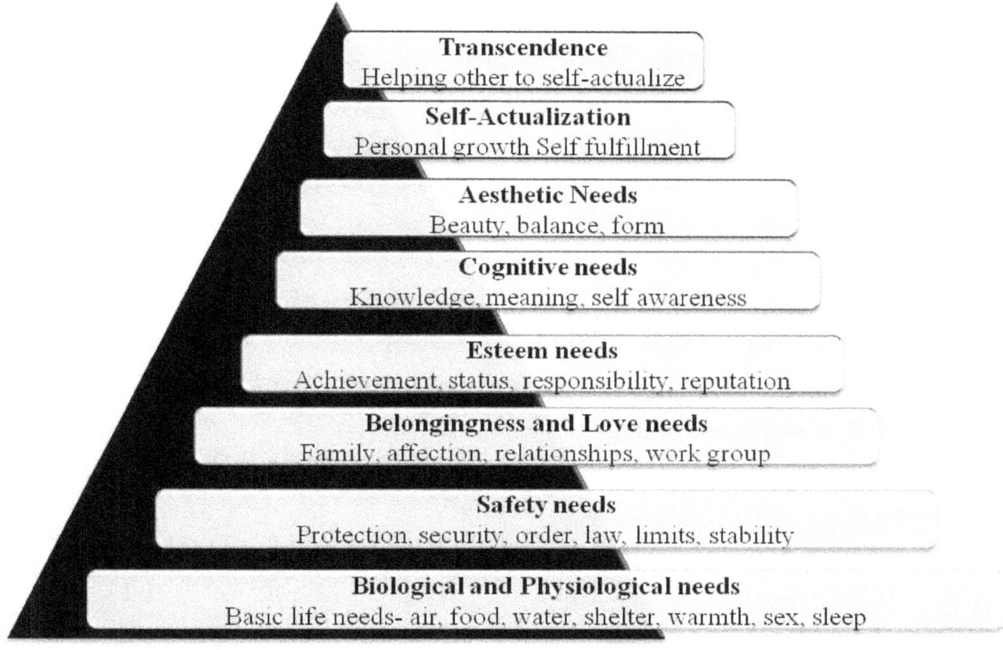

5) Answer D:

The analysis of a Pareto diagram evaluates categories that represent the greatest frequency of cases. It evaluates the greatest number of incidents, not necessarily severity. In this example from *Safety Metrics 2nd Edition*, the frequency of injuries were classified according to the body part affected. Over this period, backs accounted for 40% of all injuries, hands 30%, arms 20%, and all other were 10%.

To construct a Pareto diagram, the category that accounted for the greatest percentage of cases is placed to the left of the diagram and remaining categories are arranged in descending order of overall percentage of injuries.

A Line is constructed that indicates the cumulative of injuries. In this chart, back and hand injuries account for 70%; while back, hand and arm account for 90%.

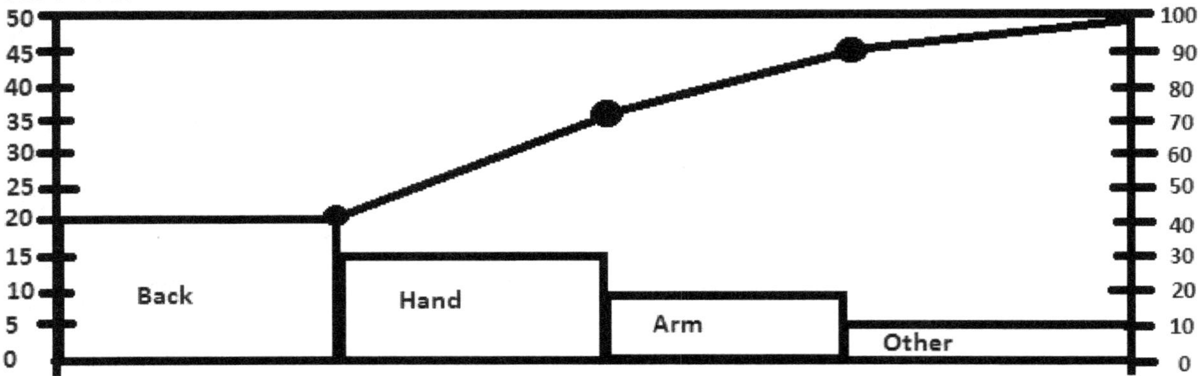

6) Answer C:

Pre-and post-testing as a measurement of the learning, the tests should cover the same areas but be phrased differently. Each pre- and post-test question item should be written for each course learning objective. For ease in assessing the course learning, you should match the question item as close as possible to the learning objectives.

7) Answer C:

Perception surveys are most often used when one is trying to find out how people understand or feel about their situations or environments. They are used to assess needs, answer questions, solve problems, establish baselines, analyze trends, and select goals. Surveys reveal what exists, in what amount, and in what context. The two main reasons why companies conduct surveys are to get feedback on past/current performance and/or to obtain information for future direction. However, they can be used far beyond just a way to gather information. They can:

- Identify gaps and provide recommendations to rectify between what is said and what is practiced
- Highlight differences between management and employees, realizing that the larger the gap, the greater the problem
- Provide an opportunity to connect and interact with employees
- Identify gaps between company's goals and its actual policies
- Serve as internal benchmarks, a measurable and quite useful means for companies to follow its own trends and progress
- Determine where current programs work and where they fall short
- Be an operational tool because responses from employees can really drive action

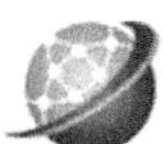

- Make employees feel that management does care what they have to say
- Encourage employees to provide feedback to management, thereby getting a sense of their role as part of the business aspects of organizations
- Encourage open communication among various organizational layers

Since almost all major companies and industries are conducting surveys, it is more important that companies be confident that the survey chosen will provide responses that will be useful to its operation. In other words, the survey must be reliable and validated. To get everyone thinking and talking about safety in the same way, it is necessary that perception surveys be conducted at all levels in a company. That is the only way true communication can begin. Administration and conduction of the survey is crucial. Confidentiality and anonymity must be absolutely guaranteed. Otherwise, respondents will not be honest, and the survey results will be essentially useless. It is only with the assurance of anonymity and confidentiality that employees will feel safe responding to questions truthfully. The perception survey results, with evidence-based recommendations, will give management a blueprint for action.

8) Answer A:

According to the National Safety Council, some of the elements of an effective safety culture are:

- The CEO must express support for safety and show it by their actions and decisions.
- The management team must consistently support safe work conditions and obtain safer materials/machines.
- The front-line supervisors need to correct behaviors as well as obtain the right equipment.
- The workers must want to be safe and work as a team.
- The union must make safety part of its role in protecting the members.

A total safety culture requires continual attention in the domains of environment, person factors and behavior. In an effective organization, line management is responsible and accountable for enforcing SH&E policies.

9) Answer C:

Some safety professionals question the lack of design and engineering influence on the accident causation model advanced by management theorists (based on behavioral aspects). However, understanding motivations for people's actions, as well as realizing how they act, affords the ability to design better and safer facilities, equipment and tools.

10) Answer C:

Most experts agree that there are two primary actions that influence behavior change the most, positive reinforcement and reinforcing the behavior as close to time of action as possible. The first step in improving behavior in an organization is to establish an ethics program to address the organization culture issues.

11) Answer A:

Frederick Herzberg in his book *Work and the Nature of Man* develops a motivation-hygiene theory. The theory attempts to explain how persons are satisfied by certain job factors while being motivated by other factors that are quite peripheral to the job being performed. Two-factor theory distinguishes between:

Satisfaction is influenced by:	Motivation is influenced by:
Money	Achievement
Status	Recognition
Relationships with Boss	Enjoyment of work
Company policies	Possibility of promotion
Work rules	Responsibility
Working conditions	Chance for growth

- **Motivators** (e.g. challenging work, recognition, responsibility) that give positive satisfaction, arising from intrinsic conditions of the job itself, such as recognition, achievement, or personal growth.
- **Hygiene factors** (e.g. status, job security, salary, fringe benefits, work conditions) that do not give positive satisfaction, though dissatisfaction results from their absence. These are extrinsic to the work itself, and include aspects such as company policies, supervisory practices, or wages/salary.

12) Answer D:

The annual performance evaluation provides an excellent opportunity to train, counsel and encourage employees. However, correcting employee shortcomings or encouraging superior performance should occur during normal daily supervision. The employee annual performance evaluations should always be based on sound, measurable objective criteria that is fully understood by both the supervisor and employee. The meeting should **never** be used as a way for the supervisor to express his or her personal feelings about the lack of potential of a worker. Providing negative comments about

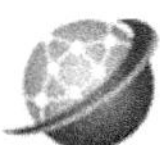

the potential for success or failure is poor practice.

13) Answer B:
Benchmarking (also "best practice benchmarking" or "process benchmarking") is a process used in management and particularly strategic management, in which companies evaluate various aspects of their business processes in relation to best practice, usually within their own industry. Benchmarking is researching other organizations methods, selecting the best techniques and applying them to your organization. This then allows companies to develop plans on how to adopt such best practice. Benchmarking may be a one-of event but is often treated as a continuous process in which companies continually seek to challenge their practices. A safety performance benchmark is like a goal. An example would be one year with no lost time injuries or illnesses at a work site. A bench mark is based on research conducted on other similar organizations and applied to your organization. Incident rates are lagging indicators (sometimes referred to as business metrics) of safety performance. Overall safety performance cannot be evaluated by historical data such as these rates and are typically poor performance indicators

14) Answer A:
An effectiveness evaluation is defined as "a determination of the extent to which program operations have contributed to achieving an objective related to accident or injury reduction. It involves (a) determining the change achieved in accident or injury involvement, (b) relating program operations to the achieved change and (c) relating the program cost to the benefit derived from what the program accomplished.

15) Answer B:
Accountability for safety performance in the superior performing companies is clearly established with line management at every level. Safety performance is one of the elements scored in the overall performance measurement system. Favorable or unfavorable results influence salaries, bonuses, and promotion potential. One of the principal indicators of management commitment to safety is the inclusion of safety performance in the performance review system. Management commitment to safety is questionable if the accountability system does not include safety performance measures that impact financially and on the promotion potential of those responsible for results. (Swartz, 2000)

16) Answer B:
The 9, 1 supervisor would be one who is interested more in production than in the interests of their employees and thus would be labeled a Dictator or organizational manager. Conversely, a 1, 9 managers might be referred to as a country club manager.

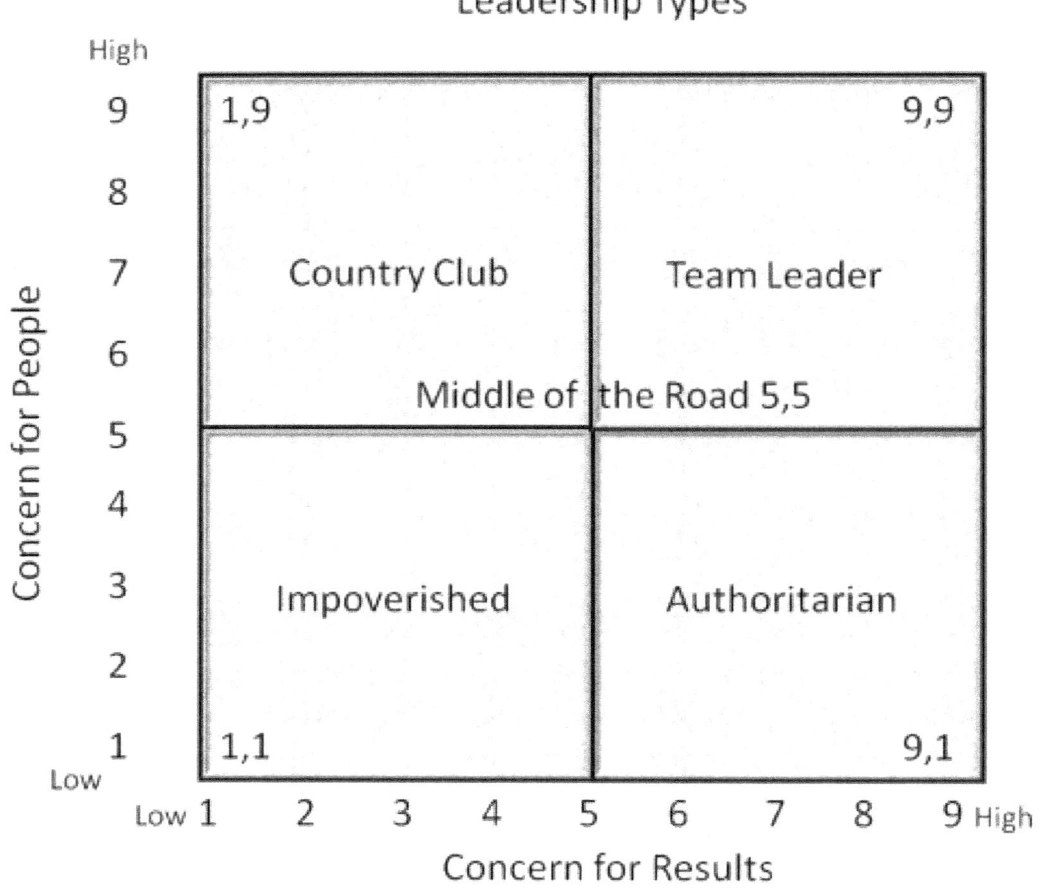

17) Answer D:
The key concepts in empowerment strategies generally include:

- Ownership. Ownership implies trust and should come with delegation of authority commensurate with the tasking. No self-directed work team is truly productive until the team members hold themselves mutually accountable.
- All contributions are valuable. It is important to value all input and, in many cases, a "try it you will like it" attitude is in order. Every idea is important to the originator.
- Everyone has value. All jobs have dignity; treat everyone with respect.

 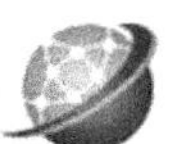

- Listen to the smallest voice. Contributions come from all corners; often the greatest offering will come from the lowest stature employee.
- Delegate authority to the lowest possible level. If employees are competent, then let them do their job. No one knows more about the of a job than the person doing it.
- Teams must own the problem. Teams must be given autonomy. If management does not trust the team, then management is the problem. Management, within reason, cannot change recommendations that come from teams.

Selection d) offers a typical bureaucratic review process that will kill the initiative of a team because it burdens them with extensive justification at many levels. Ownership is a simple concept, but hard to accomplish. Any attempt at nitpicking, over supervision, rephrasing, rearranging etc. will undermine the empowerment through ownership strategy.

18) Answer D:
The purpose of adopting OHSAS 18001 health and safety management system is to maintain continuous improvement. If the management system finds a significant reduction in the company's safety performance, it should indicate a comprehensive management review of specified items causing the reduction.

19) Answer D:
Most experts agree that depicting the bottom line cost will have the greatest impact on upper level management. This may be done by comparing losses to budgets or future estimated cost impacts and how they will impact unit costs.

20) Answer A:
The insurance industry uses EMR for workers' compensation insurance as a means of determining equitable premiums. These rating systems consider the average incident losses for a given firm's type of work and amount of payroll and predict the dollar amount of expected losses due to work-related injuries and illnesses. All 50 states, DC, Guam and Puerto Rico have worker's compensation laws. If you have an experience modifier greater than 1, you have above average losses and a less than standard performance. The EMR is based on the last 3 years loss history, not including the previous year.

Study References for SMS Exam

Many of these publications can be ordered online via websites such as asse.org; nsc.org; Amazon.com; Barnesandnoble.com; etc. By comparison price shopping, some good deals on these books may be found.

The purpose of our self-study workbook is to give study effort direction. This workbook effectively narrows down the enormous amount of test material which must be mastered. Knowing what to study is not enough. Candidates must also study the **right** material, specifically, the right reference material. Finding the right books from which to study is probably the most important single element in developing a personal study plan. It is imperative to take some time and do it correctly.

The Board of Certified Safety Professionals (BCSP) provides a pamphlet entitled "Examination Guide". In this pamphlet several pages are devoted to the subject of study references. There are numerous references listed for the SMS Examination. However, the following references have proven to be most valuable to safety professionals studying for this exam:

1) ANSI/ ASSE Z10 (2012). *American National Standard for Occupational Health & Safety Management Systems.* Des Plaines, Illinois: American Society of Safety Engineers.
2) ASSE/ANSI (2009). American National Standard: Criteria for Accepted Practices in Safety, Health and Environmental Training. ANSI Z490.1-2009. Des Plaines, IL: ASSE, 2009.
3) BCSP. (2017). *Complete Guide to the SMS®*. Champaign, IL: Author.
4) Brauer, R. (2006). *Safety and Health for Engineers* (2nd ed.). Hoboken, New Jersey: Wiley & Sons Inc.
5) Hagan, P.E. (2009). *Accident Prevention Manual: Administration & Programs* (13th ed.). Printed in the United States of America: National Safety Council Press.
6) Hagan, P.E. (2009). *Accident Prevention Manual: Engineering & Technology* (13th ed.). Printed in the United States of America: National Safety Council Press.
7) Haight, J.M. (2012). *The Safety Professionals Handbook: Management Applications* (2nd ed.). Des Plaines, Illinois: American Society of Safety Engineers.
8) Haight, J.M. (2012). *The Safety Professionals Handbook: Technical Applications* (2nd ed.). Des Plaines, Illinois: American Society of Safety Engineers.
9) Hill, D.C. (2014). *Construction Safety Management and Engineering*

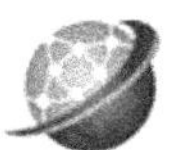

(2nd ed.). Des Plains, Illinois: American Society of Safety Engineers.

10) International Organization for Standardization (ISO). (2011). Guidelines for auditing management systems (ISO 19011:2011).

11) International Organization for Standardization (ISO). (2011). Risk Management Principles and Guidelines (ISO 31000:2011).

12) International Organization for Standardization (ISO). (2011). Environmental management Systems (ISO 14001:2011).

13) Keys, C. (2014). *Consultants Business Development Guide*, Park Ridge, Illinois: American Society of Safety Engineers.

14) Manuele, F. (2003). *On the Practice of Safety* (3rd ed.). Hoboken, New Jersey: Wiley & Sons Inc.

15) Petersen, D. (2003). *Techniques of Safety Management: A Systems Approach*. (4th ed.). Des Plaines, Illinois: American Society of Safety Engineers.

16) Plog, B.A. (2012). *Fundamentals of Industrial Hygiene* (6th ed.). Printed in the United States of America: National Safety Council Press.

17) Snyder, D.J. (2014). *Pocket Guide to Safety Essentials* (2nd ed.). Printed in the United States of America: National Safety Council Press.

18) Snyder, D.J. et al. (2014). *The Hazardous Materials Management Desk Reference* (3rd ed.). Bethesda, Maryland: Alliance of Hazardous Materials Professionals.

19) Snyder, D.J. (2018). *How Safety Professionals Influence decision makers*. Unpublished Doctoral dissertation, The University of Arkansas.

20) Strahlendorf, P. (2004). Professional Ethics for the Health and Safety Professional. June 2004 ASSE Conference proceedings Las Vegas.

www.ingramcontent.com/pod-product-compliance
Lightning Source LLC
Chambersburg PA
CBHW081803200326
41597CB00023B/4133
* 9 7 8 1 2 8 4 3 2 2 9 8 9 *